369 0026891

KU-875-860

A Manual for
Blood
Conservation

LIBRARY
ACCESSION No. 8989
CLASS WB 356
SUB
BLOOD TRANSFUSION

MONKLANDS HOSPITAL
AIRDRIE ML6 0JS

Edited by
Dafydd Thomas
John Thompson
Biddy Ridler

tfm Publishing Ltd, Castle Hill Barns, Harley, Nr Shrewsbury, SY5 6LX, UK.
Tel: +44 (0)1952 510061; Fax: +44 (0)1952 510192
E-mail: nikki@tfmpublishing.com; Web site: www.tfmpublishing.com

Design and layout: Nikki Bramhill
Front cover image courtesy of Image, c/o Dene Bank Design, Havant
Copyright © 2005 tfm publishing Ltd.

ISBN 1 903378 24 9

The entire contents of *A Manual for Blood Conservation* is copyright tfm publishing Ltd. Apart from any fair dealing for the purposes of research or private study, or criticism or review, as permitted under the Copyright, Designs and Patents Act 1988, this publication may not be reproduced, stored in a retrieval system or transmitted in any form or by any means, electronic, digital, mechanical, photocopying, recording or otherwise, without the prior written permission of the publisher.

Neither the authors, the editors nor the publisher can accept responsibility for any injury or damage to persons or property occasioned through the implementation of any ideas or use of any product described herein. Neither can they accept any responsibility for errors, omissions or misrepresentations, howsoever caused.

Whilst every care is taken by the authors, the editors and the publisher to ensure that all information and data in this book are as accurate as possible at the time of going to press, it is recommended that readers seek independent verification of advice on drug or other product usage, surgical techniques and clinical processes prior to their use.

The authors, editors and publisher gratefully acknowledge the permission granted to reproduce the copyright material where applicable in this book. Every effort has been made to trace copyright holders and to obtain their permission for the use of copyright material. The publisher apologizes for any errors or omissions and would be grateful if notified of any corrections that should be incorporated in future reprints or editions of this book.

Printed by Gutenberg Press Ltd., Gudja Road, Tarxien, PLA 19, Malta.

Tel: +356 21897037; Fax: +356 21800069.

Contents

		page
Foreword	Marcela Contreras	vii
Chapter 1	Blood Letting and Blood Giving - A History of Blood Transfusion *Michael JG Thomas*	1
Chapter 2	Transfusion Transmitted Infections *David Howell, John Barbara*	13
Chapter 3	National Inventories *Judith Chapman*	23
Chapter 4	Who Needs Transfusion? *Brian McClelland*	35
Chapter 5	Practicalities and Tips: How to Do it *June Frankpitt, Biddy Ridler*	45
Chapter 6	The Role of the Hospital Blood Bank *Joan Jones, Bill Chaffe*	57
Chapter 7	Acute Normovolaemic Haemodilution *Richard J Telford, Jonathan M Hall*	65
Chapter 8	Intra-operative Cell Salvage *John F Thompson*	75
Chapter 9	Surgical Methods to Minimise Blood Loss *John V Taylor, Francesco Torella*	87
Chapter 10	Anaesthetic Methods to Minimise Blood Loss *Philip MS Dobson*	101
Chapter 11	Pharmacological Approaches *Roger Cordery, David Royston*	113

Chapter 12   Postoperative Cell Salvage   123
                 Andrew Hamer

Chapter 13   Transfusion Triggers in Surgical   133
                 and Critically Ill Patients
                 Timothy S Walsh

Chapter 14   Management of Transfusion on the Ward   149
                 Magnus Garrioch

Chapter 15   Haemostasis for Surgeons and Anaesthetists   165
                 Denise O'Shaugnessy, Timothy Farren

Chapter 16   Transfusion Triggers in Medical   179
                 Patients with Chronic Anaemia
                 Clare Taylor

Chapter 17   Assisting Patients who Refuse Transfusion   189
                 Paul M Stevenson

Chapter 18   Consent and Refusal: The Competent Adult   203
                 Sheila AM McLean

Chapter 19   Treating Children   213
                 Sarah Joanne Elliston

Chapter 20   Mismatching Errors in the   225
                 Blood Transfusion Process
                 Margaret O'Donovan

Chapter 21   Audit and Clinical Governance   241
                 Richard Lee, Bruce Campbell

Chapter 22   The Hospital Transfusion Team   251
                 Dafydd Thomas

Chapter 23   Education in Blood Transfusion   265
                 and the Transfusion Practitioner
                 Karen Shreeve, Elizabeth S Pirie

Chapter 24   Regulatory Framework   277
                 Virge James, Dorothy Stainsby

Contributors

John Barbara MA MSc PhD FIBiol FRCPath, Microbiology Consultant to the National Blood Authority, National Transfusion Microbiology Department, National Blood Service, London, UK

Bruce Campbell MS FRCP FRCS, Professor & Consultant Surgeon, Royal Devon and Exeter Hospital, Exeter, UK

Bill Chaffe CSci FIBMS, Transfusion Co-ordinator, East Kent NHS Trust, Ashford, UK

Judith Chapman FIBMS MBA, Manager, Blood Stocks Management Scheme, London, UK

Marcela Contreras MD FRCPath FRCPEdin FRCP, Professor of Transfusion Medicine, RFUCHMS, Director of Diagnostics, Development & Research, National Blood Service, UK

Roger Cordery FRCA, Fellow, Anaesthesia, Harefield Hospital, Harefield, UK

Philip MS Dobson BSc MB ChB FRCA, Consultant Anaesthetist, Northern General Hospital, Sheffield, UK

Sarah Joanne Elliston MA (Cantab), LLM, Barrister (non-practising), Lecturer in Medical Law, University of Glasgow, Glasgow, UK

Timothy Farren BSc(Hons) AIBMS, Clinical Research Fellow, Southampton University Hospital NHS Trust, Southampton, UK

Jane Frankpitt SRN, Head Phlebotomist, Royal Devon and Exeter Hospital, Exeter, UK

Magnus Garrioch MB ChB (Birm) FRCA FRCP (Glasg.), Consultant in Anaesthesia and Intensive Care, Part-time Senior Lecturer, Southern General Hospital & University of Glasgow, Glasgow, UK

Jonathan M Hall B Med Sci (Hons) BM BS MRCP FRCA, Specialist Registrar, Royal Devon and Exeter Hospital, Exeter, UK

Andrew Hamer MB ChB MD FRCS(Orth), Consultant Orthopaedic Surgeon, Northern General Hospital, Sheffield, UK

David Howell BSc PhD SRCS, Head of Surveillance, Transfusion Microbiology, National Transfusion Microbiology Department, National Blood Service, London, UK

Virge James DM (Oxon) FRCPath MBA, Consultant Haematologist, National Blood Service, Sheffield, UK

Joan Jones CSci FIBMS, Manager Hospital Transfusion Practitioner Team, Welsh Blood Service, Cardiff, UK

Richard Lee BSc FRCP FRCPath, Consultant Haematologist, Royal Devon and Exeter Hospital, Exeter, UK

Brian McClelland MB ChB ND Linden FRCP(E) FRCPath, Consultant Haematologist, Scottish National Blood Transfusion Service, Edinburgh, UK

Sheila AM McLean LLB M Litt PhD LLD (Abertay, Dundee), LLD (Edinburgh) FRSE FRCGP FRCP(Edin) FRSA, International Bar Association Professor of Law and Ethics in Medicine, Director, Institute of Law and Ethics in Medicine, University of Glasgow, Glasgow, UK

Margaret O'Donovan RN PGdip MIHM, Risk Manager, Royal Free Hospital NHS Trust, Hampstead Heath, London, UK

Denise O'Shaughnessy FRCP FRCPath DPhil, Consultant Haematologist, Southampton University Hospital NHS Trust, Southampton, UK

Elizabeth S Pirie MSc BSc PG Cert RGN, Transfusion Nurse Specialist / Education Co-ordinator, Effective Use of Blood Group, Scottish National Blood Transfusion Service, Edinburgh, UK

Biddy Ridler MB ChB, Clinical Blood Conservation Co-ordinator, Royal Devon and Exeter Hospital, Exeter, UK

David Royston FRCA, Consultant Anaesthetist, Harefield Hospital, Harefield, UK

Karen Shreeve RGN RM FETC, Hospital Services Transfusion Practitioner, Welsh Blood Service and Swansea NHS Trust

Dorothy Stainsby FRCP FRCPath, Consultant Haematologist, National Blood Service, Newcastle upon Tyne, UK

Paul M Stevenson Chairman, Hospital Liaison Committee for Jehovah's Witnesses, Exeter, UK

Clare Taylor MB BS PhD FRCP MRCPath, Consultant in General Haematology and Transfusion Medicine, Royal Free Hospital, London and National Blood Service, North London, UK & Honorary Senior Lecturer, Royal Free and University College Medical School, London, UK

John V Taylor MB ChB, FRCS (Ed), Specialist Registrar, Vascular Surgery, University Hospital Aintree, Liverpool, UK

Richard J Telford BSc (Hons) MB BS FRCA, Consultant Anaesthetist, Royal Devon and Exeter Hospital, Exeter, UK

Dafydd Thomas MB ChB FRCA, Consultant in Intensive Care and Anaesthesia, Morriston Hospital, Swansea, UK

Michael JG Thomas MA MB BChir FRCP Edin LMSSA DTM&H, Clinical Director, The Blood Care Foundation, Fleet, Hants, UK

John F Thompson MS FRCSEd FRCS, Consultant Surgeon, Royal Devon and Exeter Hospital, Exeter, UK & Council member, British Blood Transfusion Society

Francesco Torella MD FRCS (Gen), Consultant Vascular Surgeon, Honorary Senior Lecturer in Surgery, University Hospital Aintree, Liverpool, UK

Timothy S Walsh BSc(Hons) MB ChB(Hons) MRCP FRCA MD, Consultant in Anaesthetics and Critical Care, New Edinburgh Royal Infirmary, Edinburgh, Scotland, UK

Foreword

The last two decades have seen a rapid and significant progression in the development of transfusion medicine as a specialty in its own right. Although allogeneic blood transfusion has never been safer from viral risks, after the realisation that HIV can be transmitted by transfusion, the perception of the public and our political masters, fed by the media, is that blood is becoming increasingly unsafe. There is the absurd and unrealistic aspiration to "zero risk" by transfusion. There is a desire to increase the number or complexity of expensive microbiological screening tests and blood component manufacturing procedures, with a justification that their introduction will improve the safety of the blood supply. Research continues to concentrate on enhancing the already high safety of blood and developments are mainly directed at convincing the public that all possible measures are being taken to decrease current and hypothetical infectious risks of transfusion to negligible levels. The tremendous preoccupation with the infectious risks of blood was considerably amplified in 1996, with the report of the first cases of variant CJD. The threatened risk of transmission of the abnormal prion of vCJD by transfusion led to the introduction of expensive measures in the UK Blood Services to protect recipients of blood and blood derivatives.

The emphasis in the prevention of transfusion transmitted infections has meant that other risks of transfusion, such as giving the wrong blood to the wrong patient, have been neglected. In addition, it is only recently that clinicians, managers and governments have taken an interest in appropriate blood transfusion, and in a serious approach to blood conservation and alternatives to allogeneic blood transfusion.

I welcome this manual wholeheartedly. It is unique in its approach and it was long overdue. There are numerous books dedicated to clinical blood transfusion, most of them with an emphasis on the laboratory aspects of immunohaematology, microbiology and blood component preparation, exalting the advantages of blood and blood component transfusion. This book is different in its approach. It is refreshing and stimulating that the editors are real users and prescribers of blood, with a long-standing interest in blood conservation and transfusion medicine in general. It is not often that we see a consultant anaesthetist, a consultant surgeon and a blood conservation co-ordinator participating actively in meetings, congresses and symposia related to transfusion medicine. We are now reaping the rewards of the interests of this amply qualified "trio", which have culminated in the publication of this very well-planned, and practical, manual. The sequence of chapters is well-structured, all written by authorities in their respective fields. This is a review of the wide-ranging aspects that matter to anybody who is genuinely interested in safeguarding blood, this precious resource, for those who really need it.

The manual will, I am sure, be an important, unprecedented addition to the library of all those prescribing and administering blood and blood components. It should also appeal to staff in blood banks and blood services, as well as to physicians and decision-makers in public health. I have no doubt that it will make a significant contribution to ensuring a sufficient and safe blood supply.

Marcela Contreras MD FRCPath FRCPEdin FRCP
Professor of Transfusion Medicine, RFUCHMS
Director of Diagnostics
Development & Research
National Blood Service, UK

Chapter 1

Blood Letting and Blood Giving - A History of Blood Transfusion

Michael JG Thomas MA MB BChir FRCP Edin LMSSA DTM&H

Clinical Director, The Blood Care Foundation

Fleet, Hants, UK

"Richard Lower, Sir Christopher Wren .... transfused humans with blood from animals as well as concoctions of ale, wine and other fluids .... "

Introduction

Man has always had a deep fascination with blood and, since earliest times, has endowed it with mystical powers and healing properties. Shedding blood has always evoked altruistic emotions, as is illustrated when Jesus said "This is my blood, which I shed for you." Language associates blood with passion, using terms such as "hot-blooded", "cold-blooded" and "bad blood". Literature frequently uses blood as an allusion to altruism as is illustrated by Henry Vth's famous speech "For he today that sheds his blood with me shall be my brother" (Figure 1).

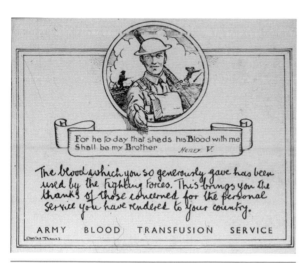

Figure 1. Blood Donor Certificate From WWII.

Historically, the needs of those wounded in war have led to many major advances in blood transfusion. The most important is the ability to draw blood in one location and transfuse it later, in another location. Another important advance was the need for meticulous planning, especially with regard to donor organisation and the logistics of blood transport and storage. On the other hand, war has not led to many direct innovations in the clinical use of blood transfusion; rather, military medicine has tended to reflect advances in civilian practice. However, the increased funding made available during war has allowed new ideas to be introduced much quicker than would have happened in peacetime.

In spite of this longstanding fascination with blood, blood transfusion is a very recent phenomenon. In the 19th century, blood transfusion was used for the treatment of disease, rather than resuscitation, and its use to combat shock only appeared in the First World War, when many techniques had already been developed in civilian hospitals.

Before the 20th century

In 1492, Pope Innocent VIII had an apoplectic stroke. His physician decided to rejuvenate him by transfusing him with blood taken from four youths. The Pope died, the youths died and nothing more was heard of the physician. By the middle of the 17th century, curious scientists, including Richard Lower and Sir Christopher Wren in England and Jean-Baptiste Denis in France, were experimenting with transfusion. Their early work was in animal-to-animal experiments, but latterly, they transfused humans with mammalian blood as well as concoctions of ale, wine and other fluids. As the majority of these transfusions proved fatal, transfusion was either banned or made illegal. Denis was tried for murder and narrowly escaped with his life.

Following this, the vogue for blood letting became prevalent. It is said that more British officers died at the Battle of Waterloo from the attentions of their physicians, who regularly prescribed blood thinning, than were killed by French bullets.

Consequently, transfusion fell into disrepute until 150 years later when, in 1818, James Blundell, a British obstetrician, performed the first successful transfusion of human blood to a patient for the treatment of postpartum haemorrhage. Using the patient's husband as a donor, he extracted a small amount of blood from the husband's arm and, using a syringe, successfully transfused the wife. Between 1825 and 1830, he performed ten documented transfusions, five of which proved beneficial to his patients. He also devised various transfusion instruments.

The earliest reported case of a transfusion in a military setting was one of a transfusion of artificial serum, composed of whey, albumin, muriate and phosphate of soda, to a soldier suffering from cholera [1]. Initially, the patient's condition improved dramatically and, although he subsequently died, the transfusion was given for what we would now consider a sound clinical reason - the replacement of fluid volume. As the 19th century came to an end, the use of cow's and goat's milk and various combinations of resuscitation fluids were replaced by saline infusions with a consequent fall in transfusion reactions.

1900 - 1914

Two major developments occurred at the beginning of the 20th century, that were to revolutionise blood transfusion. The first was the discovery in 1900, by Karl Landsteiner, of the ABO blood group system (Figure 2) [2]. Unfortunately, his work was not widely publicised and so numerous alternative blood-grouping nomenclatures came into use, including two numeric ones [3,4]. The use of confusing blood-grouping systems persisted until the advent of World War II finally led to the universal adoption of the ABO system [5]. The second was the independent development by Alexis Carrel [6] and George Crile [7] of methods by which a donor's artery could be attached to a recipient's vein; the so-called "direct" method. Although they initially attracted more interest than Landsteiner's work, the shortcomings associated with both techniques stimulated research for better "indirect" methods. These new techniques initially involved the use of syringes coated with wax [8], but were superceded by the discovery by Agote [9], Hustin [10] and Lewisohn [11] that citrate was a safe and effective anticoagulant

---

Abdruck aus dem
Centralblatt f. Bakteriologie, Parasitenkunde u. Infektionskrankheiten.
I. Abteilung.
Herausgeg. von Dr. O. Uhlworm in Cassel. — Verlag von Gustav Fischer in Jena.
XXVII. Bd. 1900. No. 10/11.

Nachdruck verboten.

Zur Kenntnis der antifermentativen, lytischen und agglutinierenden Wirkungen des Blutserums und der Lymphe.

[Aus dem pathol.-anat. Univ.-Institute des Prof. W e i c h s e l b a u m
in Wien.]

Von Dr. **Karl Landsteiner** in Wien.

1) Das Serum gesunder Menschen wirkt nicht nur auf tierische Blutkörperchen agglutinierend, sondern öfters auch auf menschliche, von anderen Individuen stammende. Es bleibt zu entscheiden, ob diese Erscheinung durch ursprüngliche individuelle Verschiedenheiton oder durch die erfolgte Einwirkung von Schädigungen etwa bakterieller Natur bedingt ist. Thatsächlich fand ich das erwähnte Verhalten bei Blut, das von Schwerkranken herrührte, besonders ausgeprägt. Es könnte diese Erscheinung mit dem von M a r a g l i a n o geschilderten Lösungsvermögen des Serums für Blutkörperchen bei verschiedenen Krankheiten zusammenhängen. (IX. Kongr. f. inn. Med. 1892.)

Figure 2. Karl Landsteiner's groundbreaking publication leading to the
the introduction of blood group serology as a science within medicine.

The First World War

Blood transfusion was first seen as a mass life-saving measure during World War I. Although the United States did not officially enter the war until 1917, American surgeons were teaching British and French doctors transfusion techniques from as early as December 1914. Direct methods needed surgical expertise to anastomose the donor's artery to the recipient's vein, and these techniques required the participation of at least three people. In addition, donors frequently lost their radial arteries and, as it was difficult under field conditions to measure the amount of blood transfused, problems arose from both under-transfusion and over-donation [12]. L Bruce Robertson [13], a Canadian surgeon who had trained before the war under Lindemann at the Bellevue Hospital in New York, supported Jeanbrau's contention that direct donation was useless in war. The introduction of citrated blood coupled with a citrate-glucose storage solution described by Rous and Turner in 1916, however, allowed an American surgeon, Captain OH Robertson, to establish the first blood "depot" in the British Army [14], where blood was stored for up to 14 days. Unfortunately, citrated blood led to numerous febrile reactions, probably caused by bacterial contamination of the distilled water used to make up the citrate solution, coupled with inadequate cleaning of the transfusion equipment [15]. These reactions were incorrectly attributed to citrate itself which fell into disrepute, and so transfusing fresh blood directly from donor to patient once again became the vogue.

The inter-war years

In October 1921, Percy Lane Oliver established the first civilian unremunerated donor panel in Camberwell, South London. When a London hospital required blood, it would contact Oliver, who kept a register of volunteers. He would then arrange for the volunteer to go to the relevant hospital. In 1926 this service became London-wide and expanded until, in 1938, 6,538 donations were arranged. In 1932, the first hospital blood depot was established in Leningrad, Russian Federation. In 1935, the International Society of Blood Transfusion was founded and in 1936, Hyland marketed the first vacuum blood collection bottle, which enabled Bernard Fantus in 1937 to set up the first hospital blood bank in the US at Cook County Hospital, Chicago. He is credited with the term "blood bank".

During the Spanish Civil War (1936-1939), Duran Jorda established a blood bank in Barcelona, and Norman Bethune, a Canadian surgeon, set one up in Madrid [16]. Both developed the concept of taking blood to the wounded rather than the wounded to the blood. However, their methods were complex and involved mixing several donations of the same group. In an attempt to prevent the growth of anaerobic bacteria, pressurised air was forced into each bottle, converting 99% of the haemoglobin to oxyhaemoglobin.

The Second World War

As the prospect of war loomed, a meeting was held at the War Office to discuss the provision of a transfusion service. The advent of the tank brought mobility to the battlefield and transformed the way in which wars were fought. The concept of a major static hospital, close to the front line, with a plentiful supply of rearward troops to act as donors, was no longer tenable. Two options were considered: the first was to blood group every member of HM Forces and issue all medical units with the equipment required to run a donor session, so that blood could be obtained where it was needed with the minimum delay; the other option was to set up an Army Blood Transfusion Service (ABTS), based on an elaborately equipped Army Blood Supply Depot (ABSD) in the UK, from which supplies could be sent to transfusion units close to the front.

The Committee decided to follow the second. Experience gained during the war, and from subsequent campaigns, has shown that, it is virtually impossible to find the time or personnel, at the height of a heavy battle, to set up a donor session. During the war, the German medical services, who had adopted the policy of "bleeding on the hoof", were constantly short of blood. This also applied to the Americans until they abandoned this practice and set up a central blood collection depot in the UK, firstly to take donations from US troops stationed in England, and subsequently, to act as a distribution centre for blood delivered from the US.

The physical link of having the donor and recipient in close proximity had been broken and the stage was set for an increase in the use of blood transfusion [17]. This could only be achieved by efficient blood collection, which is illustrated by donation records of the time. In 1938, the last complete year before World War II, the Greater London Red Cross donor panel arranged 6,538 donations, whereas by June 1940, the *monthly* figure for blood donations taken by the ABTS alone had risen to 113,500.

To enable these targets to be met, a sophisticated donor call-up and re-call system was set up, which differed very little from that practised within the present day National Blood Service. A donor panel of some 5,000 had been recruited before the outbreak of hostilities, but this soon increased to 100,000, and exceeded half a million by the end of the war. The techniques used would be recognised today. Local organisers encouraged friends and work colleagues to attend donor sessions, celebrities were asked to donate and national heroes provided endorsements.

1945 to date

After the war, it was realised that the structure which had proved so successful for blood collection should be preserved and so, in 1946, the National Blood Transfusion Service was founded in England and Wales and in 1947, the American Association of Blood Banks was formed.

Components

The introduction, in 1950, by Carl Walter and WP Murphy Jr. of the plastic blood collection bag enabled a number of earlier scientific discoveries to be combined and the practice of component therapy to be developed. In 1940, Edwin Cohn, Professor of Biological Chemistry at Harvard Medical School, developed the cold ethanol fractionation process for breaking down plasma into components, which enabled albumin, gamma globulin and fibrinogen to be used in clinical practice.

Fractionation has provided new therapies for the treatment of disorders such as haemophilia and immune deficiency diseases but probably the most important benefit has been the prevention of Rhesus Haemolytic Disease of the Newborn (HDN). In 1939, Karl Landsteiner (who, with Philip Levine, in 1925, had already described the M, N and P systems), Alex Wiener, Levine and RE Stetson discovered the Rhesus blood group system. Soon after this, HDN was described, but until 1967, when Rhesus immune globulin was commercially introduced, the only treatment had been exchange transfusion. Now, prevention was possible.

The new plastic collection bags not only allowed plasma to be separated from the cellular components so that it could be used for fractionation, but platelets could be produced, which revolutionised the treatment of leukaemia and other malignancies. The remaining red cells could then be better presented in an optimal additive solution [18].

The major contribution that the military has made to transfusion medicine since World War II has been cryopreservation. The Berlin Airlift and the start of the Cold War brought the realisation that, whilst it was possible to stockpile military and medical supplies, this was not true of blood, which at that time had a shelf-life of only three weeks. This gave impetus to the search for a simple, inexpensive method for cryopreserving erythrocytes. In 1949, Polge proposed glycerol as a cryoprotectant for freezing spermatozoa, and in the following year, Smith [19] reported the successful cryopreservation of red cells, also using glycerol. In 1962, the Ministry of Defence (MoD) set up the Blinde project in conjunction with the US Office of Naval Research. The initial aim was to use polyvinylpyrrolidone (PVP) as a cryoprotectant. PVP was found to be unsuitable and so in 1966, trials were conducted with glycerol using the method of Krijnen and Rowe [20]. Stocks of glycerolised red cells were laid down in Germany and at the ABSD. Whilst the US forces used -80° mechanical freezers, the British used lower concentrations and stored in the vapour phase of liquid nitrogen at -150°. Unfortunately, the need to wash the red cells prior to transfusion imposed an unacceptable delay, so in 1969, work was started on an alternative cryoprotectant - hydroxy-ethyl starch (HES). The technique was patented in 1992 [21].

Transfusion transmitted diseases

When Percy Oliver set up the transfusion service in the 1920s, donors completed a health questionnaire, underwent a brief medical examination and were tested for syphilis. Methods of preventing transfusion transmitted diseases (TTDs) progressed no further until testing for hepatitis B surface antigen was introduced in 1971, although Beeson had published his description of transfusion transmitted hepatitis (serum jaundice) in 1943.

The emergence of acquired immune deficiency syndrome (AIDS) in the early 1980s highlighted the need for better screening of potential donors. In 1985, the first human immunodeficiency virus (HIV) antibody test was introduced. Since then the techniques of donor interviewing have been greatly improved and tests for human T-cell leukaemia virus (HTLV), hepatitis C (HCV) and HIV p24 antigen were introduced in 1989, 1990 and 1996 respectively. Using the advances made in genetic engineering, Nucleic Acid Amplification Testing for HIV and HCV was introduced in 1999.

Autologous transfusion

The impetus for the development of autotransfusion came from the US in the early 1970s in response to the growth of coronary artery surgery, although the first recorded use of the technique was by James Duncan, in Edinburgh, in 1886. Roche and Stengle in 1973, reported a survey of transfusion practices in US institutions performing cardiopulmonary bypass surgery [22]. They found the average blood use was eight units per case and predicted the continued growth of this form of surgery, suggesting that cardiac surgery would soon consume the majority of the United States' allogeneic blood resources.

HIV and the introduction of the Paul Gann Blood Safety Act gave an impetus to Pre-operative Autologous Donation (PAD), but it was soon realised that this was an expensive procedure, which, in most cases, was not cost-effective and which resulted in surgery being performed on anaemic patients.

The future

Will blood transfusion become an anachronism? Although a true genetically engineered artificial blood is probably at least 30 years away, oxygen carrying resuscitation fluids will probably be clinically available within the next five years. If a screening test for variant Creutzfeldt Jakob (vCJD) is developed, the donor base may be diminished by anything from 5% to 20%. Blood conservation techniques, such as better pre-operative preparation of patients, anaesthetic techniques, lowering the transfusion threshold and bloodless surgery will all need to be instituted as a matter of course.

Key Summary

◆ 1900 Landsteiner described the ABO blood group system.

◆ 1914-16 Agote, Hustin and Lewisohn developed methods for anticoagulating blood.

◆ 1917 Oswald Robertson set up the first blood depot.

◆ 1939 Donor collection and organisation instituted.

◆ 1940 Cohn fractionation.

◆ 1950 Introduction of plastic collection bags.

◆ 1967 Introduction of Rhesus immune globulin.

◆ 1985 HIV screening test developed.

References

1. Renwick W. Transfusion in a case of cholera. *Dublin Medical Press* 1854; 31: 258-9.
2. Landsteiner K. Über Agglutinationserscheinungen normalen menschlinchen Blutes. *Weiner Klinik Wochensctire* 1901; 1: 5-8.
3. Jansky J. Haematologicke, studie u. psychotiku. *Sb Klin Praze* 1907; 8: 85-139.
4. Moss WL. Studies on isoagglutinins and isohemolysins. *Johns Hopk Hosp Bull* 1910; 21: 63-70.
5. Gunson HH, Dodsworth H. Fifty Years of Blood Transfusion. *Transfus Med* 1996; 6 (Suppl 1):1-88.
6. Carrel A. The surgery of blood vessels. *Johns Hopk Hosp Bull* 1907; 18: 18-28.
7. Crile G. The technique of direct transfusion of blood. *Ann Surg* 1907; 46: 329-32.
8. Kimpton AR, Brown JH. A new and simple method of transfusion. *JAMA* 1913; 6: 117-8.
9. Agote L. Neuvo procedimiento para la transfusion de sangre. *Annals of the Institute of Clinical Medicine* 1915; 1.
10. Hustin A. Principé d'une nouvelle methode de transfusion. *Journal of Medicine (Brussels)* 1914; 2: 436.
11. Lewisohn R. Blood transfusion by the citrate method. *Surg Gyn Obs* 1915; 21: 37-47.
12. Chevassu M. "Emile Jeanbrau (1873-1950)". *Bulletin de l'Academie de Médicine* 1950; 134: 420-5.
13. Robertson LB. Transfusion of whole blood. *BMJ* 1916; July 8th: 38.
14. Robertson OH. A method of citrated blood transfusion. *BMJ* 1918; 27th Apr: 477-9.
15. Lewisohn R, Rosenthal N. Prevention of chills following the transfusion of citrated blood. *J Am Med Assoc* 1933; 100: 466-9.

16.   Franco A, Cortes J, Alvarez J, Diz JC. The development of blood transfusion: the contributions of Norman Bethune in the Spanish Civil War (1936-1939). *Can J Anaesth* 1996; 43(10): 1076-8.

17.   Thomas MJG. The Army Blood Supply Depot. In: Gunson HH, Dodsworth H, Eds. *Transfus Med* 1996; 6 (Suppl 1): 65-71.

18.   Högman CF, Akerblöm O, Hedlund K, *et al.* Red cell suspensions in SAG-M medium. *Vox Sang* 1983; 45: 217-23.

19.   Smith AU. Prevention of haemolysis during freezing and thawing of red blood cells. *Lancet* 1950; ii: 910.

20.   Krijnen HW, Kuivenhoven ACJ, de Wit JJFrM. The preservation of blood cells in the frozen state. In: *Modern problems of blood transfusion*. Speilman W, Seidl S, Eds. Gustav Fischer, Stuttgart, 1970.

21.   Thomas MJG, Parry ES, Nash SG, Bell SH. A method for the cryopreservation of red blood cells using hydroxyethyl starch as a cryoprotectant. *Transfusion Science* 1996; 17(3): 385-96.

22.   Roche JK, Stengle JM. Open heart surgery and the demand for blood. *J Am Med Assoc* 1973; 225(12): 1516-21.

Chapter 2

Transfusion Transmitted Infections

David Howell BSc PhD SRCS

Head of Surveillance, Transfusion Microbiology

John Barbara MA MSc PhD FIBiol FRCPath

Microbiology Consultant to the National Blood Authority

National Transfusion Microbiology Department, National Blood Service, London, UK

"The risk associated with transfusion transmitted infections is usually only a small part of the overall risk."

Introduction

The potential risks to recipients of blood transfusion are similar to and often less than risks from other activities that are acceptable to the public such as playing football or travelling by car (Figure 1). It is still necessary to appraise the recipients of blood and its components of the risks, alternatives and any potential risk from these alternatives. When discussing the risks with the patient it is necessary to consider the particular circumstances of the recipient. Different advice might be given depending on the severity of their illness and potential life span, i.e. the balance between risk and benefits.

Safe donated blood is an expensive resource and there has been much work on development of effective alternatives. These include cell salvage and pre-operative autologous donation/transfusion which are discussed elsewhere. It is not part of the remit of this chapter to discuss infectious risks to staff arising from using these techniques. Hospital staff should be aware that blood donors are a highly selected and tested population and their donated blood is much less likely to be infectious for human immunodeficiency virus (HIV), hepatitis B virus (HBV) or hepatitis C virus (HCV) than the general hospital population. There will be a much greater risk from a needle-stick accident involving the patient than there would be from a needle-stick accident involving donated blood.

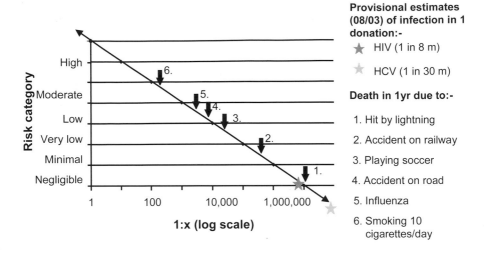

Figure 1. Risk from transfusion relative to other risks *(personal communication from K Soldan to J Barbara).*

What makes a microbial agent important to blood safety?

Any risk will depend on which blood component is involved as some agents are associated with particular components (human T cell leukaemia virus [HTLV] and cytomegalovirus [CMV] are associated with white cells). The main factors predisposing an agent to transfusion transmission are:

- Presence in blood.
- Persistence. Some organisms such as hepatitis A virus (HAV), have a viraemic phase but it is relatively short, and thus any risk of transmission is small, often sub-clinical. The donor is effectively symptomless (potential donors who feel unwell tend not to donate).
- Significant of the associated morbidity/mortality. If an agent is not pathogenic (eg. CMV in *immuno-competent* recipients), testing is unnecessary.
- Prevalence and incidence in the recipient population. If the majority of the population are already infected then there would be an argument for screening recipients and offering vaccination, if available.

There are also practical considerations:

- Assays must be affordable within the context of the overall health budget.
- The performance of the assay must be compatible with the requirements of mass, rapid microbial testing.
- The assay time must be considerably less than the shelf-life of the blood product.

Which agents are relevant to transfusion?

The significance of these agents will vary geographically and each country should assess their own priorities and ascertain the relevant significance of the agents of concern in their own particular context.

Viruses

- HBV might be automatically included as a significant risk for all countries. However, in future, this might not be the case in a country with a policy of universal post-natal HBV screening and vaccination, or with a high prevalence of hepatitis B infection such that most of the population will have been infected by the time they are adults. Specific policies would then be needed for younger recipients.

Other viruses for which most countries test are:

- HCV.
- HIV 1 and 2 (with various subtypes of HIV1).

Other viruses that are sometimes included in testing programs are:

- HTLV. Japan was one of the first countries to introduce screening because of a high incidence in the population.
- CMV is a risk to immunocompromised patients, eg. low birth weight neonates, bone marrow transplant patients. It is usual for these patients to receive blood screened for CMV antibody. Although not

proven by prospective studies, leucodepletion is likely to provide levels of safety equivalent to screening.

♦ West Nile Virus (WNV) is transmitted by mosquitoes. The UK Blood Services dealt with this potential threat to safety by excluding prospective donors who had visited the US during the mosquito season. To reduce unnecessary exclusion of donors it is planned to perform Nucleic Acid Testing (NAT) for WNV where a donor has reported a visit to the US during the relevant season.

Other viruses are known to be transmitted by transfusion, but only infrequently or with low pathogenicity for most recipients, eg. HAV, parvovirus B19.

Bacteria

The only bacterium for which specific screening is implemented is *Treponema pallidum* (syphilis). Syphilis was the first routine transfusion microbiology screen to be introduced. There has been discussion about its cost/benefit but the screening is unlikely to be withdrawn because of the perception that it is a "life-style marker".

Haemovigilance schemes continue to report morbidity and mortality associated with contamination by other bacteria. Although the number of bacterial transmissions are low, they are considerably higher than acute viral reactions. Interventions to reduce bacterial risk are at last becoming routinely implemented.

Bacterial contamination of a blood donation can be either endogenous or exogenous.

♦ Syphilis would be an example of endogenous infection. Other endogenous bacterial infections are not generally a problem for the transfusion service because the potential donor will feel unwell and will not donate. However, some transmissions of *Yersinia enterocolitica* from red cells (often nearing the end of their shelf-life) have been reported.

♦ The pattern of exogenous contamination is changing. There have been improvements in manufacturing and processing, (eg. the withdrawal of water baths to warm/thaw blood) leading to fewer "pinhole" type failures and associated contamination with organisms such as *Pseudomonas*. More common is the identification of skin contaminants arising from inadequate arm cleansing prior to venepuncture to obtain the blood donation. This has lead the National Blood Service in England to investigate different procedures for arm cleansing and also to introduce diversion of the first 20ml of the donation so that the skin bacteria contaminating the venepuncture needle are flushed away into a pouch separate from the blood collection bag.

Parasites

The importance of parasites with regard to transfusion safety depends on location but risks are changing with greatly increased global travel. Several parasitic diseases are potentially transmissible by transfusion, eg. malaria, toxoplasmosis, babesiosis, leishmaniasis. Prevention, in a non-endemic area, of transmission of parasitic disease by transfusion is achieved by exclusion from donation for a suitable period. The main problem is malaria; in the UK, current policy is to use an exclusion period together with an assay for release of blood donated by individuals who may have been exposed to malarial infection.

Prions

Two issues relating to prions and blood safety have received recent media coverage:

♦ A suspected case of variant Creutzfeldt-Jakob disease (vCJD) caused by transfusion has been reported * [1]. In 1996, before the introduction of leucodepletion, a patient in the UK aged 62 was

---

* Since preparation of this chapter, a second suspected case has been reported.

transfused with five units of red cells at the time of surgery. One of the units had been donated by a 24-year-old individual who developed symptoms of vCJD three years and four months later. Six and a half years after the transfusion the recipient started to show symptoms of vCJD and died 13 months later. The donor would therefore have been infectious three years before symptoms developed with an incubation period for transfusion transmitted disease of six years. The chance of the disease in the recipient being due to diet is 1:15,000 to 1:300,000. Following this case, from the 5th April 2004 the UK Blood Services have excluded the recipients of transfusion from blood donation.

♦ The first reported case of bovine spongiform encephalopathy (BSE) in a cow in the US (that had been imported from Canada) with the possibility of material from this animal entering the human food chain. This single case will not affect the UK's decision to source plasma from the US.

Other emerging infections

WNV, severe acute respiratory syndrome (SARS), human herpes virus 8 (HHV8), TT virus (TTV), SEN virus (SEN-V) and GB virus C have all been suggested as a threat to the safety of the blood supply. Consensus opinion is that some of these agents are not a significant risk. However, it is without doubt that dozens of new infectious diseases are likely to emerge [2], and that some of these emerging infections will pose a threat to transfusion safety. It is for this reason that efforts to improve transfusion safety will probably be directed towards pathogen inactivation and donor selection rather than donation testing.

Any additional testing introduced to improve the safety of the blood supply will have an associated cost, not just in purchasing and performing the assay but also in handling the inevitable false positive reactions. False positive donations involve a direct, associated cost (reference testing, contacting the donor, etc.), but more importantly, will exclude blood from hospital shelves. In most instances in the UK's low-risk population, only a small proportion of "reactive" donor samples prove to be positive.

Residual risk

The risk to the recipients of blood donation will depend on several factors and will be variable in different countries. For a given agent the factors are:

♦ Numbers of infected individuals in the general population.
♦ Efficiency of donor selection, i.e. numbers of infected individuals in the donor population.
♦ The rate of new infections.
♦ Immunity in recipients.
♦ Efficiency of donation testing:

- Testing errors. This is unlikely because of the use of process control.
- Assay failures. In 1996, it was reported that an HIV assay from a reputable manufacturer had failed to detect seven samples that were positive.
- Falsification of results. In 1997, it was reported that the staff of a major blood centre in the US were falsifying test results to enhance their remuneration.

♦ Supplementary tests added to improve detection such as a polymerase chain reaction (PCR); usually for HCV, sometimes for HIV and, rarely, for HBV, HIV p24, anti-HBc, neopterin, alanine amino transferase (ALT).
♦ Bacterial screening for release of product.
♦ Pathogen inactivation/reduction including filtration/leucodepletion. A Medline search using these two words produced 348 entries between 1996 and 2003 and almost half of these were published in the last two years. This is a most important area of research not only for reducing and possibly preventing new and emerging threats but also, significantly, for bacterial infections.

The following do not provide any direct input to blood safety but should be linked into a feedback mechanism designed to improve the efficiency of the testing:

♦ Haemovigilance schemes. In the UK, the Serious Hazards of Transfusion (SHOT) scheme directly assesses the residual risk of acute, symptomatic complications.

◆ Statistical control for the testing process and active/efficient quality control schemes.

Blood safety in the UK is further complicated because, following HCV litigation, blood is now regulated by the Consumer Protection Act 1987. It is important that blood safety must have adequate financial resources available.

It is obviously unethical to carry out formal transmission experiments studying the infectivity of the blood supply. However, some information has been obtained from retrospective studies on the recipients of HCV-infected blood. It could be assumed that similar work will be done following the introduction of any new screening test. The introduction of HTLV screening in the UK in 2002 has led to a review of previous recipients, which may provide information on the efficiency of leucodepletion for increasing transfusion safety.

The current safety of the blood supply is such that prospective studies are no longer feasible because of the large numbers of transfused units that need to be followed to produce meaningful results. One of the last studies in the UK was reported by Regan *et al* [3], who followed the recipients of 20,000 units of red cells between 1990 and 1995. No transfusion infection was identified. It is now necessary to use complex statistical methods to measure blood safety. These methods will rely on assumptions with wide margins of error. In the UK, Soldan [4] reported an estimated frequency of infectious units entering the blood supply to be 1:260,000 for HBV, 1:8 million for HIV and 1:30 million for HCV. The highest and lowest estimates for HBV differed by a factor of 13. Studies from other countries are compared in Table 1.

Table 1. Estimated residual risk per donation.

	England 1993-2001 Soldan [4]	US window period Schrieber [5]	Italy 1996-2000 Velati [6]	Spain 1997-99 Alvarez [7]
HBV 1:	260,000	63,000	-	74,000
HCV 1:	30 million	103,000	127,000	149,000
HIV 1:	8 million	493,000	435,000	513,000

Conclusions

Blood transfusion in the developed world is safe but never completely without risk. Risks are greater in developing countries but the costs of improvements in safety need to be considered in relation to the availability of resources within the overall budget. It is likely that the risk from bacterial contamination and from new/emerging agents will mean that a greater importance is given to pathogen inactivation.

It is without doubt that in the developed world the current risk of infectious complications following transfusion is minimal compared with the risks associated with the overall transfusion process.

Key Summary

◆ There will always be a risk associated with blood transfusion.

◆ The biggest risk will be due to clerical/identification errors.

◆ The risk associated with transfusion transmitted infections is usually only a small part of the overall risk.

◆ The magnitude of this risk will depend on local circumstances.

◆ It is important to monitor new/emerging pathogens.

◆ Alternative interventions to testing (such as pathogen reduction) merit serious consideration.

References

1. Llewelyn CA, Hewitt PE, Knight RSG, Amar K, Cousens S, Mackenzie J, Will RG. Possible transmission of variant Creutzfeldt-Jakob disease by blood transfusion. *Lancet* 2004; 363: 417-421.
2. News Round Up. *BMJ* 2004; 328: 186.

3.   Regan FAM, Hewitt PE, Barbara JAJ, Contreras M. Prospective investigation of transfusion transmitted infection in recipients of over 20,000 units of blood. *BMJ* 1999; 320: 403-406.

4.   Soldan K, Barbara JAJ, Ramsey ME, Hall AJ. Estimation of the risk of hepatitis B virus, hepatitis C virus and human immunodeficiency virus infectious donations entering the blood supply in England 1993-2001. *Vox Sang* 2003; 84: 274-286.

5.   Schreiber GB, Busch MP, Kleinman SH, Korelitz JJ. The risk of transfusion transmitted infections. *N Engl J Med* 1996; 334: 1685-1690.

6.   Velati C, Romano L, Baruffi L, Pappalettera M, Carreri V, Zanetti AR. Residual Risk of transfusion-transmitted HCV and HIV infections by antibody-screened blood in Italy. *Transfusion* 2002; 42: 989-993.

7.   Alvarez M, Oyonarte S, Rodriguez PM, Hernandez JM. Estimated risk of transfusion-transmitted viral infections in Spain. *Transfusion* 2002; 42: 994-998.

Further reading

1.   Caspari G, Gerlich WH, Gurtler L. Pathogen inactivation of cellular blood products - more security for the patient or less? *Transfusion Medicine and Haemotherapy* 2003; 30: 261-263.

2.   Dzik WH. Transfusion Safety in the Hospital. *Transfusion* 2003; 43: 1190-1199.

3.   Glyn SA, Kleinman SH, Wright DJ, Busch MP. International application of the incidence rate/window period model. *Transfusion* 2002; 42: 966-972.

4.   Wagner SJ. Transfusion-transmitted bacterial infection: risks, sources and interventions. *Vox Sang* 2004; 86: 157-163.

5.   Yomtovian R. Bacterial contamination of blood: lessons from the past and road map for the future. *Transfusion* 2004; 44: 450-159.

Chapter 3

National Inventories

Judith Chapman FIBMS MBA

Manager, Blood Stocks Management Scheme, London, UK

"There is a fine balance between supply and demand for blood - it is a freely given resource which should be managed and used carefully."

Introduction

It has been estimated that over 75 million units of blood are donated world-wide every year [1]. Ensuring maintenance of the blood supply is a primary goal of blood services who rely on the good will of voluntary donors for the supply of blood. The voluntary nature of the donation emphasises the fragile nature of the supply and the associated requirement for effective inventory management across the supply chain.

The factors that impact upon the blood supply chain include: the unpredictable nature of the supply due to reliance on volunteer donors, distribution logistics, and stock management practice across the supply chain.

The blood supply

One of the major challenges for blood services is maintaining the donor base. Volunteer donors are the source of the blood supply chain. However, despite recruitment efforts the donor base is falling in many countries. In England and North Wales, although blood donation is advertised and encouraged, the number of active donors has been shrinking and the average donation frequency of whole blood donors is declining [2]. Only 3%

of adults are currently blood donors and 50% of these give 75% of donations. A further 6% of donors lapse each year. In the US, it has been estimated that approximately 12.6 million units of whole blood are collected from approximately eight million volunteer donors, with approximately 3% of the population donating an average of 1.6 times per year [3].

The low number of donors results in blood services often experiencing problems in maintaining the supply during public holiday periods, particularly at Christmas and New Year, Easter and May public holidays which often fall close together, and the summer holiday months. In addition, safety concerns and associated increased testing have resulted in the loss of donors through deferral and disqualification. Depending on the country, the blood supply has also been affected by donor deferral, due to increased foreign travel and the associated risk of malaria and other emergent diseases, such as West Nile virus. In the UK, recently introduced precautionary measures have led to the exclusion of donors who have been previously transfused, with an estimated loss of approximately 3.3% of donors and 52,000 donations. In 2002, the US introduced donor deferral for individuals who had travelled or resided in the UK or other parts of Europe, because of the perceived risk of variant Creutzfeldt Jakob disease (vCJD). Of 9800 surveys distributed to donors in the US, 7405 were returned and analysed and gave a deferral rate of 3.5%. The most common reason for deferral was military service at a US military base in Europe, followed by residence in Europe for longer than five years [4]. The fragility of the supply has shifted the focus of blood services away from donor recruitment to recruitment conversion and donor retention. They have commissioned studies exploring donor demographics and psychographics, and use the information obtained to focus on donor retention initiatives and to target individuals in donor marketing campaigns. Initiatives being developed to try to increase retention include appointment systems and the use of postal pre-donation questionnaires.

Red cell demand

From 1992 to 2000 there was a steady increase in the demand for red cells. Since then, demand in England and North Wales has fallen year on year for the last three years (Table 1).

Table 1. Number of red cell units issued by the National Blood Service by year April 2001-March 2004.

Year	Number of red cell issues (millions)
April 2001 - March 2002	2.206
April 2002 - March 2003	2.186
April 2003 - March 2004	2.157

Demand is difficult to predict due to a number of factors, not least the very nature of healthcare. Tools such as environmental scanning, modelling and trending can be used to try to forecast demand more accurately. The National Blood Service (NBS) in England and North Wales uses projections identified by a demand planning group (DPG), which regularly prepares short- and medium-term demand projections. The group bases its figures on monthly calculations of the average number of red cells and components issued on a working day and on a weekend/public holiday. External factors such as initiatives to improve the appropriateness of red cell transfusions are also taken into consideration. Demand forecasting for the year together with target inventory levels are used to calculate an annual projected collection figure, which then forms the basis for session planning. Quarterly meetings of the DPG monitor progress against plan and make adjustments if necessary.

Factors that may increase demand include:

- Population demographics.
- Advances in medical procedures and trauma care.
- Increased commitment and spending to Health Services by governments.

A recent study carried out in the North of England showed that the average age of a patient receiving a unit of blood was 62.7 years. Using data from the study and population predictions, it was estimated that annual red cell demand would increase by 4.9% in 2008 [5]. The mapping of the human genome will increase knowledge of diseases such as cancer and may result in more aggressive treatments that may require increased transfusion support. Fall in demand may be attributable to a number of reasons including:

- The increasing price of a red cell unit.
- Increased use of conservation techniques such as intra-operative cell salvage.
- More appropriate use of blood.
- Lower Hb trigger levels.
- Increased use of therapeutic agents such as erythropoietin (EPO) and aprotinin.

Inventory management

As far back as 1975, Cohen and Pierskella [6] applied techniques of management science and mathematical inventory theory to construct a model for management strategies for a regional blood bank, describing control policies for the inventory system.

Inventory levels

In blood services, appropriate inventory levels are key to effective inventory management. The inventory level in a blood centre will depend upon the type of centre, the hospitals that it serves, or whether it is part of a national or independent blood service. Blood services have the advantage that they can move blood around the country or to other centres belonging to the service, to satisfy times of glut or shortage, or equipment failure. In the NBS a national stock manager uses age peak algorithms to determine movements around the blood centres. This ensures that if any one centre is holding excess numbers of red cell units that are older, the potential use of these units can be maximised by moving some of the units from the peak to other NBS centres.

Blood service inventory levels should take into account the need to balance the requirement to meet demand from hospitals, against the age at issue and time expiry wastage. Potential national crises may also influence stock holding with a requirement to hold sufficient inventory to cope with national emergencies. Hospital inventory levels are influenced by similar factors. The ability to meet clinical demand and the need to cope with emergencies must be balanced against potential time expiry wastage which incurs a cost to the hospital. Hospital inventory levels will also depend on the hospitals' clinical specialties, the distance from the blood centre and transport arrangements.

Monitoring inventories

Effective inventory management techniques such as "just-in-time" (JIT) match supply to demand. JIT techniques used in the industrial and commercial business sector are suitable for some areas of healthcare, but do not translate well to the blood supply system, mainly because of the risk of an inventory shortage. Insights into the whole blood supply chain lead to an increase in the understanding of blood inventory management [7]. Blood services generally have detailed knowledge of the donor element of the supply chain, including collections, processing, testing and wastage. There is minimal knowledge of the hospital end of the supply chain. In April 2001, the NBS and the hospitals it serves, established the Blood Stocks Management Scheme (BSMS) to increase understanding of the whole blood supply chain including blood stock management in hospitals. Data collection is based on a SQL database, in which data are stored on red cell and platelet issues, inventory, wastage and shelf-life. Data are entered onto the BSMS database either through downloads from computer systems or manual data entry via the BSMS website (www.bloodstocks.co.uk). Web deployment gives flexibility in terms of multi-user access for the input and extraction of data and information. Using the web, standard reports can be generated automatically from the data in real time, allowing tactical use of the information on a day-to-day basis by all participants.

Participating hospitals and all NBS blood centres can access real time graphical displays. The graphs show data and an average of other participants' data, which is anonymised. Participants also have the opportunity to benchmark performance against other users, for example, those with similar blood usage. These graphical displays act as a driver for change since hospitals and blood centres can compare their performance to their peers.

The relationship between blood service and hospital inventories

The BSMS has shown that the number of days of red cell stock in the blood service inventory has a direct impact on the level of wastage in both the NBS and hospitals (Figure 1).

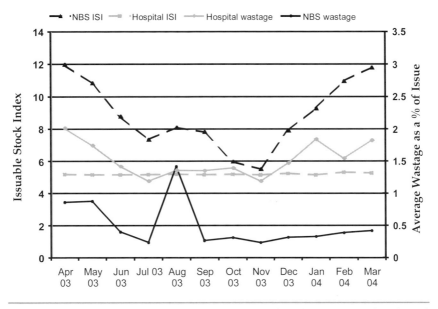

Figure 1. The relationship between NBS red cell inventory level and supply chain wastage. (ISI = Issuable stock index).

The primary reason for this is the change in the age of the red cells at issue, which is associated with changes in the stock level. The inventory held in the hospitals is very stable at approximately five days and so any variation in inventory level is absorbed by the blood service and results in ageing of the stock profile. Higher blood service red cell stock levels lead to hospitals receiving blood that has a reduced shelf-life. This means that units do not have sufficient days left to circulate through the reserved/unreserved stock loop enough times to be transfused and are eventually time-expired. The impact of the stock ageing varies between hospitals because the number of times a unit can be expected to pass through the reserved/unreserved stock loop is different, but in general, hospital wastage reacts predictably to changes in stock level.

Effective management of the hospital inventory

The Blood Stocks Management Scheme carries out regular inventory practice surveys on stock management practice including crossmatch reservation periods, ordering practice including who places the order and how the order is calculated, dereservation times, training in stock management and the use of maximum surgical blood order schedules. The results of these surveys have enabled the scheme to build up a picture of stock management practice and relate it to stock levels and wastage from the BSMS data.

Red cell ordering Standard Operating Procedure

A survey carried out in 2001 identified that of 76 respondents, 72% had a documented Standard Operating Procedure (SOP) for placing red cell orders [8]. Of those respondents that did not have a SOP, 81% had a benchmark stock level for each blood group. Four respondents had neither a SOP nor a benchmark stock level.

The analysis of the relationship between having a SOP and the standard deviation in Issuable Stock Index (ISI) suggested a lower variability for those having a SOP ($p < 0.1$). This relationship held for all blood groups except O Neg, B Pos, and group AB units ($p > 0.2$).

The preferred method of estimating how many red cell units to order was "manual calculation" with 46% of orders produced this way. Thirty-six percent of orders were calculated by visual review and 19%, almost one in five, were using computer software programs to determine orders.

Crossmatch reservation period

When crossmatch reservation periods were examined it was found that 71% of respondents reported a 48-hour reservation period (Table 2) [9].

Table 2. Frequency and percentage of each crossmatch reservation period.

Crossmatch reservation period	Frequency	Percent
24 hours	12	15.8
48 hours	54	71.1
72 hours	10	13.2

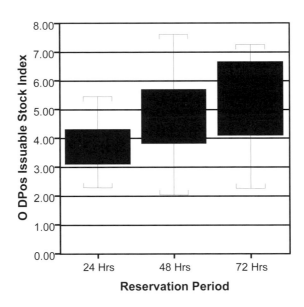

Figure 2. Box plots of median O DPos ISI for each reservation period.

The median ISI equating to days of stock held in the inventory was used as an estimate of average stock holding and was calculated for each hospital over the period 02/04/01 to 31/08/02. O Pos had the lowest ISI and the least variation; therefore, O Pos was used as an indicator of a hospital's stock level. A box plot of O DPos ISI for each of the three reservation periods, 24, 48 and 72 hours (Figure 2) showed a clear increase in the median ISI for successively increasing reservation periods. Analysis suggested a weakly significant effect of reservation period on median O DPos ISI ($p<0.1$). Further analysis indicated a significant linear trend ($p<0.05$) and a significant difference between a 24-hour period and longer reservation periods ($p<0.05$), but no significant difference between 48 hours and 72 hours ($p>0.3$). For an optimum inventory level a 24-hour reservation period is preferable, although it may not be possible for every hospital to adopt this policy as local conditions such as the presence of off-site facilities, will inevitably influence practice.

Electronic issue

A survey of the blood stocks management scheme 2002 registration questionnaires identified 27 hospitals using electronic issue (Table 3) [10].

Table 3. Number of hospitals using electronic issue.

Blood usage category	Number of hospitals using electronic issue
High usage (>11,000 red cell units per annum)	14
Moderate usage (6,000-11,000 units per annum)	11
Low usage (<6,000 units per annum)	2

The issue, stock, and wastage data from these hospitals were analysed and compared to peer hospitals not using electronic issue (EI).

Since December 2002, EI "high-usage" hospitals have consistently received less issues than non-EI users. Although no data are currently available on when hospitals started using EI, this increasing difference is likely to reflect more "high-usage" hospitals starting to use EI. Hospitals using EI are able to reduce their red cell issues because less red cell units are tied up in crossmatch fridges and available issuable stock can be used more efficiently.

Analysis of the average "high-usage" hospitals' red cell ISI, indicates that those hospitals using electronic issue hold less days worth of stock than those hospitals not using EI. The average OPos ISI for EI users was consistently below the level for the non-users. The difference has become more pronounced since December 2002.

Analysis of red cell wastage in "high-usage" hospitals indicates that those using electronic issue waste, on average, less than those hospitals not using EI. In 18 months between October 2001 and September 2003, wastage by EI users was up to seven units less per month than non-users.

The findings demonstrate that the use of electronic issue can lead to reduced red cell issues, a lower inventory level and reduced wastage. The use of electronic issue can be at least as safe as serological crossmatching provided that all the procedures outlined in the British Committee for Standards in Haematology guidelines are followed [11,12].

Other approaches to improving inventory management

In the 2002 IPS, 20% of participants indicated that they had installed a stock-expiring notice board positioned in a prominent place to inform staff of units that were approaching time expiry. In the 2003 IPS, 27% of hospitals indicated that they had entered into a stock share relationship with another hospital, mainly to reduce wastage. Fifty-two percent of hospitals had employed a transfusion practitioner.

Conclusions

In the blood supply chain there is a dynamic relationship between supply, daily demand, inventory levels and wastage. A commitment to active management of each of the elements of the supply chain will ensure effective use of this freely given resource.

Key Summary

Blood centres can ensure optimum utilisation and minimum wastage by:

◆ Holding appropriate inventory levels.
◆ Improving donor retention.
◆ Enhancing demand planning.

Effective hospital inventory management practice includes:

◆ The presence of a stock ordering SOP.
◆ A 24-hour crossmatch reservation period.
◆ Electronic issue.
◆ Stock management training.
◆ A stock sharing relationship with another hospital or Trust.
◆ Use of a stock-expiring notice board.
◆ Presence of a transfusion practitioner.

References

1. Goodnough LT, Shander A, Brecher ME. Transfusion medicine; looking to the future. *Lancet* 2003; 361: 161-169.
2. Reynolds E, Wickenden C, Oliver A. The impact of improved safety on maintaining a sufficient blood supply. *Transfusion Clinique et Biologique* 2001; 8: 235-239.
3. Davey RJ. Recruiting blood donors: challenges and opportunities. *Transfusion* 2004; 44: 597-601.

4.   Murphy EL, Connor D, McEvoy P. Blood donors and blood collection. Estimating blood donor loss due to the variant CJD travel deferral. *Transfusion* 2004; 44: 645-650.

5.   Wells AW, Mounter PJ, Chapman CE. Where does blood go? Prospective observational study of red cell transfusion in north England. *BMJ* 2002; 325: 1-4.

6.   Cohen MA, Pierskella WP. Management policies for a regional blood bank. *Transfusion* 1975; 15: 58 - 67.

7.   Chapman JF, Hick R. Monitoring the nation's blood supply. *Transfusion* 2003; 11: 1639.

8.   The Blood Stocks Management Scheme Inventory Practice Survey, 2001. www.bloodstocks .co.uk.

9.   The Blood Stocks Management Scheme Spotlight on Electronic Issue, 2003; www.bloodstocks.co.uk.

10. BCSH. Guidelines for blood bank computing. *Transfus Med* 2000; 10: 307-314.

11. BCSH. Guidelines for compatibility procedures in haematology and blood transfusion laboratories. *Transfus Med* 2004; 14: 59-73.

Acknowledgments

The author wishes to thank Rob Hick and Clive Hyam for the data analysis and all the participants in the Blood Stocks Management Scheme.

Chapter 4

Who Needs Transfusion?

Brian McClelland MB ChB ND Linden FRCP(E) FRCPath
Consultant Haematologist
Scottish National Blood Transfusion Service, Edinburgh, UK

"Transfusion has risks but bleeding to death is fatal."

Good blood management: understanding the harm and benefit

Receiving a blood transfusion should be safe for the patient, as the chance of an adverse event due to the transfusion will constitute only a small part of the total risks of the episode of care. However, there are still risks in being transfused. The media generally confuse the risks that we have now virtually removed - hepatitis B, human immunodeficiency virus (HIV) and hepatitis C - with unknown or unquantifiable "new" risks, like variant Creutzfeldt Jakob disease (vCJD). The events that are in reality more likely to harm a blood recipient, such as getting the wrong unit of blood, tend to attract less attention. A patient who receives his or her own, rather than a donor's blood avoids the risks of an allogeneic tissue transfer. "Getting your own back" may be attractive, but things can still go wrong with autologous pre-donations or blood salvage transfusions. Other blood conserving measures could also prove to have their own risks.

Much more important is to know when and how likely it is that a transfusion may do the patient some good. Where there is uncertainty, we should be extremely wary about exposing the patient to any risks associated with a transfusion, even if these are quite small. Transfusion is important or essential for some patients, but we regularly prescribe blood components without a clear understanding of the probability that they will provide a clinical benefit.

Why do we believe in transfusion?

Massive blood losses in surgery or trauma may be managed by collecting and re-infusing the patient's own blood. However, even in this obvious indication for transfusion the traditional belief in the life-saving properties of transfusion are founded on practice, very different from today's. The bleeding patient will receive red cells, largely free of plasma, with the white cells removed, typically stored for about two weeks before it is infused and perhaps supplemented with plasma and platelet concentrate [1, 2]. In the past, whole blood, often collected freshly from donors, would be used and there would be no access to fluids, drugs and equipment now available for resuscitation. While it is reasonable to expect that blood will continue to be a mainstay of the management of major haemorrhage, the effectiveness of today's blood components should continue to be critically evaluated in the context of developments in the management of haemorrhage, for example the use of novel agents such as recombinant factor VIIa (see Chapter 11).

Good blood management

Terminology referred to in this chapter is defined in Table 1. There are many ways in which the need for transfusion can be reduced or avoided. This is good blood management, defined as: management of the patient who is at risk of transfusion so as to minimise the need for allogeneic transfusion and improve the probability of a good clinical outcome.

Put another way, it is good medicine to avoid using donor blood when you can avoid it, but don't put the patient at risk for a principle. Transfusion has risks, but bleeding to death is fatal (Table 2).

Does transfusion work?

For many aspects of transfusion practice, the belief in the effectiveness of blood is not supported by adequate clinical trials. Either the trials are too small to allow conclusions to be drawn, or the completion of large, well-designed randomised controlled trials has shown little or no evidence of benefit from giving blood.

Table 1. Terminology of blood products.

Blood product	Therapeutic substance prepared from human blood.
Blood component	Platelets Red cells Fresh frozen plasma Cryoprecipitate White cells
Plasma derivative	Plasma proteins prepared from human plasma under pharmaceutical manufacturing pooled conditions, (coagulation factors, immunoglobulin, albumin, etc).
Allogeneic blood	Blood, or blood components from another, genetically different individual of the same species.
Autologous blood	An individual's own blood: collected before a planned operation, or recovered during or after an operation for re-infusion with or without further processing.

These definitions are used by the WHO and in the EU Blood Directive 2002/98/EC, "Setting standards of quality and safety for the collection, processing, storage and distribution of human blood and blood components" and also, in the UK Handbook of Transfusion Medicine. www.transfusionguidelines.org.uk

Table 2. Good blood management.

Manage the patient who is at risk of transfusion so as to:

♦ minimise the need for allogeneic transfusion, and
♦ maintain or improve the probability of a good clinical outcome, but
♦ don't forget: transfusion has risks, but bleeding to death is fatal.

Fresh frozen plasma

The UK uses about 300,000 units of fresh frozen plasma (FFP) each year [3]. Stanworth *et al* [3] reviewed 57 clinical trials of FFP. Only three of these were capable of giving a conclusion on effectiveness: the first was on the use of FFP to prevent neonatal intracranial haemorrhage and showed no benefit; the second trial showed no benefit in acute pancreatitis; and the third provided evidence that in treating thrombotic thrombocytopaenic purpura, plasma exchange with FFP was more effective than infusion of FFP. For other situations, none of the trials identified were adequate to allow conclusions to be drawn about effectiveness. A major trial of FFP in anticoagulant reversal is only now starting in the US and a planned UK trial of FFP in surgery remains on the drawing board [4, 5].

Red cells

About 2,500,000 units of red cells are supplied to UK hospitals annually. Studies in the UK and Europe [6, 7, 8, 9] indicate that about half are used for surgery and about 5% are used for patients in intensive care [10, 11].

Hill *et al* [12] systematically reviewed clinical trials comparing liberal or conservative regimes for red cell transfusion in such patients. The most substantial evidence comes from a single large randomised trial in critically ill patients in intensive care [13]. This showed that clinical measures of outcome (survival and organ failures) were lower in patients managed with contrasting regimes - either lower haemoglobin levels maintained with the use of less transfusion, or higher haemoglobin levels, involving more transfusion. Smaller trials included in the review were inadequate to provide reliable conclusions, though the reviewers suggested that these also showed a trend towards better outcomes when less blood was used.

A recent randomised controlled trial of red cell transfusion for neonates in critical care has also shown a lack of benefit from red cell transfusion [14]. These and other studies challenge the basis of current guidelines for transfusing red cells in critical illness or surgery.

Fresh or stored?

A recent study [15] assessed the effect of transfusion in intensive care unit (ICU) patients who were transfused at haemoglobin levels below 80g/L. Patients were randomised to receive blood stored for less than five days or more than 25 days. There was no difference between the effect of fresh and stored red cells on any measures of systemic or regional oxygenation. Furthermore, in neither group was there evidence that oxygenation improved following transfusion, raising questions about the physiological rationale for transfusion consistent with the findings in the trials mentioned previously.

Albumin or crystalloid?

The utility of some blood plasma derivatives is also in question. The first well-designed large randomised controlled trial of human albumin [16] has shown that it offers no benefit over saline infusions in resuscitation. The study showed an excess of deaths in patients with brain injuries who received albumin, but the authors emphasise that this could be a chance observation. This study resolves a debate that has raged since 1999 [17] and suggests that the choice of resuscitation fluid should be based on clinical experience, availability and cost.

Patients' age and medical conditions

Blood transfusion is used more commonly as patients get older [7]. Conditions that cause anaemia, impaired coagulation or platelet disorders increase the need for blood component replacement. There is some evidence to suggest that patients with coronary artery disease, whilst undergoing ICU treatment, benefit from the use of a rather higher threshold for red cell transfusion and that prognosis after myocardial infarction might be better if a low admission haemoglobin is raised by transfusion [18]. Some studies also suggest that patients with heart failure may have an improved prognosis and reduced drug requirements if maintained at a higher level of haemoglobin with erythropoietin [19]. Whether the same effect would be observed in such patients by increasing the haemoglobin level with red cell transfusion has not been investigated.

Table 3. Illustrative list of blood-saving interventions that make sense.

Before planned surgery

♦ Assessment at a pre-admission clinic.
♦ Correcting treatable anaemia.
♦ Stopping anticoagulants and antiplatelet drugs if safe to do so.
♦ Erythropoietin and/or iron.
♦ Pre-donation of blood, with haematinics with or without erythropoietin.
♦ Minimising the blood taken for laboratory samples.

During surgery

♦ Losing less blood through optimal surgical and anaesthetic technique
♦ Keeping the patient warm.
♦ Using measured haematocrit or blood loss as a guide to red cell replacement.
♦ Using rapid haemostasis testing to guide blood component replacement.
♦ Antifibrinolytics (aprotinin or tranexamic acid) to reduce bleeding in selected cases.
♦ Intra-operative cell salvage.

Postoperatively

♦ Postoperative blood salvage.
♦ Use of a protocol to trigger re-exploration at a specified level of blood loss.
♦ Use of a protocol to guide when haemoglobin should be checked.
♦ The use of a protocol stating blood transfusion thresholds and targets is associated with lower use of blood. Restricting blood prescribing to designated staff.
♦ Minimising the blood taken for laboratory samples.

Note that not all of these have been formally proven to be effective in reducing the need for allogeneic transfusion.

Variations in transfusion in elective surgery

In elective surgery, there are big differences in the use of blood for the same operations done by different surgical teams, which can only be partly explained by features of the patients treated [20]. This is typical of situations in which there is uncertainty about the effectiveness of a treatment and probably reflects differences in attitude among clinical teams or individual practitioners. Those who believe it is important to minimise transfusion are likely to place more emphasis on surgical haemostasis, and on use of other blood-conserving measures covered in this book. They are more likely to transfuse less frequently, although the precise reasons for using less blood may be difficult to pin down.

Many teams now routinely perform major surgical procedures with little or no transfusion. This is achieved by a commitment to good blood management, with attention to all the details of the patient's care that can help to avoid the need for transfusion. Specific blood-sparing procedures, such as blood salvage play a part in good blood management, but clinical trials show that these techniques have little effectiveness when trialled by teams who already manage their patients with little transfusion [21].

Perisurgical interventions to reduce the need for blood

There is a wide range of interventions that may help to conserve blood, although in many cases, there is inadequate evidence to prove that what is a good idea makes a difference in day-to-day practice. Table 3 illustrates the range of measures that may, individually or in combination, help to reduce the need to transfuse.

Key Summary

◆ For some patients with major bleeding, transfusion remains a life-saver.

◆ When a patient is at risk of death from blood loss, the priority is to provide blood in sufficient quantities and quickly.

◆ It is irrelevant to be pre-occupied with very small risks of transmitting an infection, but highly relevant to avoid further harm to the patient that would result from administering an incompatible unit of blood.

◆ The use of transfusion for similar patients having similar operations still varies widely among clinical units. This probably is a reflection of:

  • different levels of emphasis on the importance of avoiding transfusion;
  • differences in the use of a range of methods that may help to reduce the need for blood;
  • an acceptance of lower or higher haemoglobin levels as the signal to transfuse red cells.

◆ Older patients are much more likely to be transfused, and are probably more at risk than the younger subject of being harmed by acute effects of either under- or over-transfusion.

References

1. Joint NIBS-UKBTS Professional Advisory Committee 2002 Guidelines for the Blood Transfusion Services in the UK, 6th edition. The Stationery Office TSO, London. www.transfusionguidelines.org.uk.

2. *Handbook of Transfusion Medicine*, 3rd edition. McClelland DBL, Ed. www.transfusionguidelines.org.uk. The Stationery Office, London, 2002.

3.   Stanworth SJ, Brunskill SJ, Hyde CJ, McClelland DBL, Murphy MF. Is fresh frozen plasma clinically effective? *British Journal of Haematology* 2004; 126: 139-152.

4.   Dzik W. Personal communication.

5.   Williamson LP. Personal communication.

6.   Vamvakas EC, Taswell HF. Epidemiology of blood transfusion. *Transfusion* 1994; 34: 464-70.

7.   Wells AW, Mounter PJ, Chapman CE, Stainsby D, Wallis JP. Where does blood go? Prospective observational study of red cell transfusion. *North England British Medical Journal* 2002; 325: 803.

8.   Mathoulin-Pelissier S, Salmi R, Verret C, Demoures B. Blood transfusion in a random sample of hospitals in France. *Transfusion* 2000; 40: 1140-6.

9.   Titlestad K, Kristensen T, Jorgensen J, Georgsen J. Monitoring Transfusion Practice - a computerised procedure. *Transfus Med* 2002: 12: 2.

10.   Garrioch M, Walsh TS, Maciver C, Lee R, McClelland DBL, for the ATICS study group. Red blood cell use in Intensive Care in Scotland (the ATICS study). *Transfus Med* 2002; 12(Suppl 1): 6.

11.   Vincent JL, Baron JF, Reinhart K, *et al*. Anemia and blood transfusion in critically ill patients. *JAMA* 2002; 288: 1499-507.

12.   Hill SR, Carless PA, Henry DA, *et al*. Transfusion thresholds and other strategies for guiding allogeneic red blood cell transfusions (Cochrane Review). In: *The Cochrane Library*, Issue 2, 2002. Update Software, Oxford.

13.   Hebert PC, Wells GF, Blajchman MA, *et al*. A multicenter, randomized, controlled clinical trial of transfusion requirements in critical care. Transfusion Requirements in Critical Care Investigators, Canadian Critical Care Trials Group. *N Engl J Med* 1999; 340: 409-417.

14.   Kirpalani H, Whyte R, Andersen C, Asztalos E, Blajchman M, Heddle N, Roberts R, for PINT Investigators. Conservative Transfusion Regimens Are Not Associated with Higher Mortality or Morbidity in ELBW Infants The Premature in Need of Transfusion (PINT) Randomized Controlled Trial, 2004.
      http://www.pas-meeting.org/2004SanFran/Abstracts/LateBreakers/Abstracts.htm#LB15.

15.   Walsh TS, McArdle F, McLellan SA, Maciver C, Maginnis M, Prescott RJ, McClelland, DBL. Does the storage time of red blood cells influence regional or global indices of tissue oxygenation in anemic critically ill patients? *Critical Care Medicine* 2004; 32: 364-371.

16.   Finfer S, Norton R, Bellomo R, Boyce N, French J, Myburgh J for the SAFE Study Investigators. The SAFE study: saline vs albumin for fluid resuscitation in the critically ill. *Vox Sang* 2004; 87 (Suppl 2): s123-131.

17.   Cochrane Injuries Group Albumin Reviewers. Human albumin administration in critically ill patients: systematic review of randomised controlled clinical trials. *BMJ* 1998; 317: 235-40.

18.   Wu WC, Rathore SS, Wang Y, Radford MJ, Krumholz HM. Blood transfusion in elderly patients with acute myocardial infarction. *N Engl J Med* 2001; 345: 1230-6.

19.   Silverberg DS, Wexler D, Sheps D, *et al*. The effect of correction of mild anemia in severe, resistant congestive heart failure using subcutaneous erythropoietin and intravenous iron: a randomised controlled study. *J Am Coll Cardiol* 2001; 37: 1775-80.

20. The Sanguis Study group. Use of blood products for elective surgery in 43 European Hospitals. *Transfus Med* 1994; 4: 251-268.

21. Carless PA, Henry DA, Moxey AJ, O'Connell DL, Fergusson DA. Cell salvage for minimising perioperative allogeneic blood transfusion (Cochrane Review). *The Cochrane Library*, Issue 3, 2004. http://www.cochrane.org/index0.htm.

Chapter 5

Practicalities and Tips: How to Do it

Jane Frankpitt SRN

Head Phlebotomist

Biddy Ridler MB ChB

Clinical Blood Conservation Co-ordinator

Royal Devon and Exeter Hospital, Exeter, UK

"Attendance at transfusion training is now mandatory for all staff involved in the transfusion pathway ...... remember, the best transfusion is no transfusion."

Introduction

The errors documented by the Serious Hazards of Transfusion (SHOT) annual report [1] continue to increase. Blood conservation requires meticulous practice in the clinical area. The provision of incorrectly labelled samples with erroneous paperwork create problems for the transfusion laboratory which enforce delays and may lead to clinical errors affecting patient care. Coupled with this, some samples may be unnecessary in the first place.

This chapter aims to address these problems and offers tips on how to take accurate blood samples for transfusion-related requests which will help to maintain a good working relationship between professionals in the laboratory and the clinical area. Other methods will be discussed to reduce the volume of blood sampled, instructions will be provided on clearly and accurately prescribing blood products and hints will be given on how to optimise communication between all those involved in the process.

Is your blood sample really necessary?

In our experience, too many unnecessary blood samples are collected from patients each day. This can cause distress and increases the risk of errors. It also wastes time and resources, particularly if the results are not reviewed and acted upon. The higher the number of blood samples the greater the risk of errors. Junior doctors are often anxious about missing a daily blood test and it is easy to write out a request form, particularly if someone else is taking the blood! They may have been instructed (whether they agree or not) to take a sample by a more senior member of staff; often when questioned they reply "my registrar told me to". Changes in work patterns brought about by the European Working Directive [2] to improve conditions have led to a change from the static medical "Firm" to a rotation of doctors between consultant-led teams. This can mean that a doctor may work with different groups of medical colleagues during the course of their appointment. In these circumstances communication is vital between the team, particularly at hand-over/change of duty. If a blood sample has been taken and/or a blood product requested there is a responsibility to review the result and act upon it. If the doctor requesting the investigation is going off-duty it is important that a colleague assumes responsibility for this task.

Guidance for pre-operative tests can be found in a hospital's pre-admission clinic protocols. In the UK, the National Institute for Clinical Excellence (NICE) has issued guidelines [3] and in addition, the Maximum (or "Agreed") Surgical Blood Ordering Schedules will help keep venepuncture and blood ordering to a minimum level.

Near patient haemoglobin testing devices, such as the Hemocue® (Figure 1) require only a fingerprick and a small drop of blood for haemoglobin analysis, thereby saving patient distress and decreasing sample

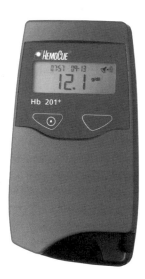

Figure 1. The Hemocue device. (courtesy of Hemocue Ltd.)

wastage. If used and maintained correctly, these devices can be very beneficial postoperatively, and in any situation where there is concern about blood loss and haemoglobin level.

Venepuncture

Venepuncture and cannulation are unpopular, sometimes painful procedures, and so staff who become skilled in these areas are much appreciated.

The aim is to obtain a valid blood sample in the correct tubes from the correct patient as painlessly as possible, hopefully leaving the vein in a good state. The process of obtaining a blood sample from a patient's vein and receiving the result can be fraught with various complications. Whilst some of the following information may seem irritatingly obvious, it is clear that the same mistakes will often occur on a daily basis.

It is helpful to look at the end results desired by the following groups involved in the chain.

- The patient - wants the blood taken as quickly and painlessly as possible, without multiple stabbings and repeat tests due to mistakes.
- The laboratory - want samples of a good quality, in the correct collection bottles filled to the appropriate level, eg. coagulation tubes. The results are only as good as the sample provided. Samples that are haemolysed or diluted with intravenous infusion fluid are unable to be analysed or will give incorrect blood values. Patients have been given inappropriate treatment as a result, i.e. wrongly transfused on the basis of an incorrect haemoglobin.
- Doctors / staff - want the results back as soon as possible in order to help diagnose and treat their patients.

Delays in the process

Patient identification

Human error in relation to patient identification is still the commonest problem [1]:

- Armband missing, illegible, or not checked.
- Patients with the same or similar name on a ward.
- Deaf or confused patients who will often answer to an incorrect name.

Check the name band if the patient is wearing one and confirm the details with them. In other situations the patient must give their name and date of birth. If the sample is for group and save or crossmatch it is essential to obtain a third point of reference - either an address or a patient identification number.

Forms

- Not filled in correctly; insufficient or incorrect patient details.
- Tests omitted or illegible.
- No ward or consultant details for laboratory to return results to.
- Incorrect form for tests requested.

Blood

- Insufficient blood for analysis.
- Blood that has haemolysed or clotted.
- Blood samples incorrectly or insufficiently labelled.
- Blood samples put in wrong tubes.

Transportation to the laboratory

- Erratic or missed collections by porters.
- Problems with pnuematic shute transportation.

- ◆ No carriers available to put samples in.
- ◆ Incorrectly packaged samples that do not meet the requirements of the postal system or courier service.

There is a growing trend for blood samples to be taken almost every day. In teaching hospitals this is partly due to the fact that new and inexperienced junior doctors are responsible for the blood requests and are often over enthusiastic, or are worried about missing something. The venesectionist, rather than the doctor, is faced with a patient who may be in pain and distressed by venepuncture, particularly if they have bad venous access and they have been in hospital for a long time. Their veins can become very bruised and traumatised, and they can also become anaemic.

Venous access is often limited by the presence of cannulas, pumps and IV infusions, so it is important to look after the few remaining veins that are accessible by carrying out careful venepuncture. Clinical reasons for not using a particular arm include: lymph node excision in the axilla usually following a mastectomy; renal fistulas; lymphoedema; and IV infusions in the same arm as the venepuncture (unless switched off)

Safety

With the increase of blood-borne diseases, particularly hepatitis and and human immunodeficiency virus (HIV), it is of the utmost importance to avoid an innoculation injury. This can be minimised by careful venepuncture technique and meticulous disposal of used sharps into appropriate containers. Never resheath needles by hand. Universal precautions must be taken. It is important to be aware of the innoculation policy in place and the procedures to follow if a needlestick injury occurs. Any skin cuts should be covered to prevent possible contamination. The use of disposable gloves is recommended although this can hamper palpation of difficult veins.

How to be successful at venepuncture

Entire books have been devoted to venepuncture and this section is only able to highlight the most salient points.

Venepuncture is purely a practical skill and the only way to become good at this is to get as much experience as possible. Taking blood from a well-filled and dilated vein is quite straightforward but unfortunately, these aren't always available! People can have bad venous access for a variety of reasons including obesity, intravenous drug abuse, chemotherapy, or very small or deep veins. Newcomers to venepuncture need to become familiar with the blood collection system used. Manufacturers provide detailed information on how to use them. There are several different types; most use a vacuum principle, which involves inserting the needle first, then applying vacuumed collection tubes. Some systems can be used like a syringe, but each sample bottle can be exchanged when full (Figure 2).

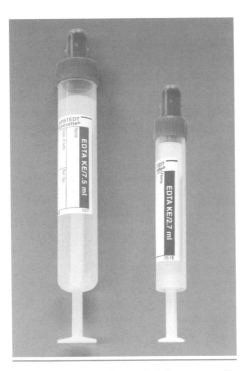

Figure 2. The S-Monovette®. (courtesy of Sarstedt AG & Co.)

Make sure that you are confident with the mechanics of attaching the sample tubes to the needle, particularly when multisampling, before you approach a patient for the first time. This inspires confidence in yourself as well as the patient! It always looks so easy until you try it for the first time. Practise on a rubber arm or even a banana until you feel confident. It really does help. There is often a tendency to push the needle in a little further with each tube change unless you are holding it firmly.

The procedure is as follows:

♦ Identify the patient correctly and explain to them what you are going to do. It is always worth spending time to select an appropriate vein by careful observation and palpation before "looking" with your needle where you expect to find a vein. Experienced patients often know where their best vein is to be found and are more than happy to tell you! Always get help to hold an arm if a patient is unable to keep it still or straight.

♦ Using a decent tourniquet makes life easier, particularly if the veins are difficult to find - patients aren't too keen on rubber gloves! Prolonged use of a tourniquet can alter the blood chemistry; for example blood for calcium estimation must be taken with the tourniquet released if possible.

♦ Assemble the equipment that you need within easy reach: needle, sample tubes, swab, tape, tourniquet and sharps bin.

♦ Skin prep, although essential for cannulation and blood cultures, is not necessary for venepuncture unless the skin is visibly soiled or the patient is neutropaenic. Topical anaesthetic cream can be used for children, or needle phobics.

♦ WASH YOUR HANDS or use alcohol rub.

♦ Use a pillow under the elbow to support and extend the arm.

The antecubital fossa is the best place for venepuncture, but the forearms and hands can also be used.

♦ Apply the tourniquet firmly about 10cm above the site and select an appropriate vein. It should feel soft and bouncy. Follow its track with your finger to ensure that you know the direction to follow when you insert the needle. Some veins travel almost horizontally. If there is nothing immediately obvious on either side, get the patient to make a fist and pump it a few times. Veins in warm limbs are much easier to find - soaking in warm water can help.

♦ Anchor the vein firmly with a finger below the site, pulling the skin taut to stabilise it during venepuncture. This is most important especially if a patient has mobile veins, and is also less painful.

♦ Remove the needle shield and insert the needle (bevel side up) into the vein at a 15% angle and fill the required tubes according to directions for the system used. If the attempt fails try repositioning the needle slightly.

NB. The order of draw is important - plain tubes without any additives must be used first to prevent possible sample contamination.

♦ When the procedure is finished, release the tourniquet, remove the needle and apply a sterile swab to the puncture site.
♦ Dispose of the needle immediately into a sharps bin.
♦ Press firmly on the vein after venepuncture. It helps prevent bruising and haematoma, conserving the vein for further access. The patient can usually be instructed to press firmly themselves for a few minutes. If they are unable to do so, the tourniquet can be used to apply pressure (don't forget to remove it!) or use your own finger to press. This may seem tedious, especially if the patient is on warfarin, but arms can be bruised and veins traumatised because this simple action was omitted.
♦ Don't ask the patient to bend their arm - this separates the skin and vein puncture sites and encourages brusing.

When you have taken the sample, label it and complete the task by the patient's side where you can be absolutely sure that the documentation is correct. This is so much safer than taking the samples back to the ward station or other public area, where you will be distracted by phones and requests for other tasks from your colleagues on the ward. It also avoids grave errors such as mixing up sample tubes or using another patient's identification details from a set of case notes lying around on the desk. Be aware that printed I/D labels can end up in the wrong patient's notes by mistake. Never ever label samples which someone else has taken and in turn, never ask anyone else to label your samples. It is essential that the request form and sample contain the following minimum patient identification:

(i) surname/family name (correctly spelt);
(ii) first name(s) in full;
(iii) date of birth (not age or year of birth)
(iv) hospital number/accident and emergency number/NHS number major incident number.

The sample should be dated, labelled and signed by the person taking it [4]. If your sample is urgent ring the blood bank and tell them! If you don't, it will be treated as "routine" by the laboratory process. Please also be absolutely clear in your request.

Is your transfusion really necessary?

You have looked at the blood results and decided that your patient may require a blood product. As we know, this course of action is not without risk. Have you:

◆ Acted on up-to-date haematological results?
◆ Reviewed the clinical condition of your patients?
◆ Considered whether any intervention is needed at all?
◆ Considered the alternatives (see Chapter11)?

If you must prescribe, do so correctly

You have carefully considered all the above, but have decided you have no choice but to prescribe a blood product. Document the reason for doing so in the casenotes. If you can honestly say, in the light of the knowledge currently available to you, that your patient needs this treatment, then should some adverse event occur you cannot be blamed for your course of action. Be guided by your hospital transfusion policy and/or ask your hospital transfusion practitioner, a member of the blood bank team or the on-call haematologist. Remember - you are not alone!

If possible, inform your patient why you believe that a transfusion is in their best interests. With access to the internet, newspapers and magazines patients are often very well-informed and may know more about the benefits and risks of transfusion than you do! If appropriate, remember to tell them about the alternatives to homologous transfusion.

In the UK, there is now a National Health Service patient information leaflet *Receiving a blood transfusion* which should be available on the wards and in clinics. Copies may be obtained from the National Blood Service Hospital Liaison Team - call 01865 440092.

Make sure that the prescription you write is the appropriate product and the correct quantity to be given to your patient over the correct length of time. It goes without saying that your writing must be legible! The name of the product should be written clearly in BLOCK CAPITALS, as for any pharmaceutical prescription.

What were the results of the transfusion?

It is important to also document the outcome of the transfusion that you have decided to prescribe.

- Did the patient benefit from blood products prescribed?
- Were there any adverse events?
- Is there a need for further transfusion?

If the patient is not actively bleeding and clinically stable, then if you can, try to adopt a "wait and see" policy. There may be artificial haemodilution, for example, particularly if the patient has undergone a long operation, which will be demonstrated by a low haemoglobin level. A diuresis in the immediate postoperative period will often raise the haemoglobin level to a more acceptable value to avoid transfusion. Similarly, a deranged clotting picture may be corrected less acutely, for example with Vitamin K instead of fresh frozen plasma.

Learn how to do it!

Attendance at transfusion teaching is now mandatory for all staff involved in the transfusion pathway. At our hospital the Department of Clinical Health Education together with the Postgraduate Medical Centre are responsible for the organisation of teaching sessions. Transfusion guidance is presented at the induction sessions for all new staff and for doctors there are twice yearly presentations at the departmental audit meetings. There is a trainer appointed for non-medical staff within each group for teaching and support.

There is also information available as a handbook [5], teaching videos, CDs and paper handouts, so there is no excuse for anyone to be ignorant about blood transfusion practice.

Key Summary

◆ Be aware of the risks in taking blood samples.

◆ Learn how to take them correctly and accurately.

◆ Ensure your sample is really necessary.

◆ Be responsible for your actions.

◆ Communicate with those involved in the care of your patient.

◆ Consider alternatives to blood products.

◆ If you must prescribe, then do so appropriately and clearly.

◆ Document your reasons in the casenotes.

◆ Don't be afraid to ask if you are unsure.

◆ Remember - the best transfusion is no transfusion!

References

1. Serious Hazards of Transfusion (SHOT) Report 2003. http://www.shot-uk.org.
2. Council Directive 93/104/EC. Official Journal of the European Community 1993; L307: 18-24.
3. http://www.nice.org.uk.
4. Working Party of the British Committee for Standards in Haematology Blood Transfusion Taskforce. Guidelines for compatibility procedures in blood transfusion laboratories. *Transfus Med* 2004; 14: 62.
5. *Handbook of Transfusion Medicine,* 3rd Edition. McClelland DB, Ed. The Stationery Office, London, 2002. http://www.thestationeryoffice.com.

Chapter 6

The Role of the Hospital Blood Bank

Joan Jones CSci FIBMS
Manager Hospital Transfusion Practitioner Team
Welsh Blood Service, Cardiff, UK
Bill Chaffe CSci FIBMS
Transfusion Co-ordinator
East Kent NHS Trust, Ashford, UK

"Communication between the blood bank and other hospital staff is a critical area."

The role of the hospital blood bank is to provide the right blood component(s) to the right patient at the right time. To be able to provide this service there are several elements which need to be considered. It is important that the patient receives support which is:

♦ Informed.
♦ Clinically indicated.
♦ Delivered in a safe manner.
♦ Timely.
♦ Cost-efficient.

Pre-transfusion testing

Every blood bank must have written policies and procedures defining their requirements for sampling, labelling and type of samples which need to be collected for performing pre-transfusion testing. Pre-transfusion testing will include the following:

♦ ABO and Rh D typing.
♦ Antibody screening to determine if there are irregular antibodies to red cell antigens.

♦ Identification of any irregular antibodies detected and an assessment of clinical significance.
♦ Comparison of current test results with historical records.
♦ Compatibility testing between recipient and donor.

This pre-transfusion testing procedure will vary from hospital to hospital. It is important that all clinicians within the organisation are aware of the time involved for the provision of transfusion support under a variety of differing circumstances. Table 1 provides a guide to the different approaches.

Table 1. The provision of transfusion support.

Procedure	Estimated time for provision of red cells	Limitations
Serological crossmatch - donor cells are tested against patient's serum/plasma	30-40 minutes	Unexpected incompatibilities
Immediate spin crossmatch - to detect ABO incompatibility	10 minutes	Not always reliable
Electronic issue - there are several essential requirements prior to this process	5 minutes	A sample must have been received by the blood bank prior to the request being made
Issue of emergency O Rh Negative units or group-specific units	5 minutes	Some patients may have irregular antibodies and may have a transfusion reaction

Role of the blood bank in communication

Communication between the blood bank and other hospital staff is a critical area. Clear policies must be in place for communicating:

◆ Routine or urgent requests.
◆ Special transfusion needs, i.e. irradiated, cytomegalovirus (CMV) negative.
◆ Clinical need in a massive transfusion episode.
◆ Clinical need for emergency O Rh Negative or group-specific units.

Role in documentation

Every blood bank must have technical Standard Operating Procedures (SOP) which ensure that staff performing pre-transfusion testing all work to the same standard. The blood bank also has a role in producing blood transfusion policies, in conjunction with the Hospital Transfusion Committee (HTC), for dissemination throughout the hospital. These policies will cover:

◆ Collection of samples, timing, labelling and type of sample.
◆ Positive patient identification.
◆ Maximum Surgical Blood Order Schedule (MSBOS).
◆ Requesting of blood components.
◆ Administration of blood.
◆ Protocols for observation of transfused patients.
◆ Use of irradiated blood components.
◆ Management of massive transfusion.
◆ Use of immunoglobulin anti-D.
◆ Transfusion triggers.
◆ Transfusion reactions.
◆ Management of major incidents.
◆ Management of blood supplies during times of national shortage.
◆ Training requirements for staff involved in the transfusion chain of practice.

Role in the HTC

The blood bank will need to provide information to the HTC in the following areas:

- Evidence that local policies are in place reflecting national guidelines.
- Evidence that the use of blood components is appropriate to clinical need.
- Wastage figures.
- Use of autologous blood.
- Education and training.
- Monitoring of adverse events and errors.
- Reviewing performance of the hospital transfusion service and the local blood centre.
- Audit activity.

Role in education and training

Staff from the blood bank are to be encouraged to participate in the education and training:

- Of all staff involved in the transfusion chain of practice.
- In the formal part of nursing and medical undergraduate courses.
- In medical and nursing induction sessions.

Role in incident reporting

The blood bank, in conjunction with the Hospital Transfusion Team (HTT) and HTC, needs to be actively involved in the investigation of adverse events and errors. Laboratory staff have long realised the importance of recording errors, working to reduce them and implementing corrective action strategies.

All blood banks must participate in the Serious Hazards of Transfusion (SHOT) reporting scheme, as recommended by the UK Health departments [1,2] and this will be mandated by the EC Directive 2002/98 on the Safety of Human Blood [3], which becomes a legal requirement in February 2005.

The SHOT scheme for the reporting of adverse events was initiated in 1996. The aim of the scheme is to educate all participants in the blood transfusion chain of practice and to act as an evidence base for blood safety initiatives, policies and guidelines. The SHOT scheme is designed to act as a national database which complements local incident reporting mechanisms rather than replacing them. Incidents that are to be reported to SHOT are:

- Incorrect blood component transfused.
- Acute transfusion reactions.
- Delayed transfusion reactions.
- Transfusion-related acute lung injury.
- Post-transfusion purpura.
- Transfusion-associated graft versus host disease.
- Transfusion transmitted infections.
- "Near miss" events.

Reporting of errors must be timely and should include notification of "near misses". Examples of near miss events to be reported include the following:

- Unnecessary or inappropriate request(s).
- Sample taken from incorrect patient.
- Incorrect interval between samples and transfusion.
- Communication regarding urgency.
- Incorrect component prescribed, i.e. irradiated.
- Incorrect component selected.
- Laboratory pre-transfusion testing errors, including clerical.
- Wastage.
- Potential for incompatible transfusion.
- Delay - hypoxia due to anaemia.

Role in multidisciplinary audit

Blood needs to be used appropriately and safely in order to conserve a finite supply for those who most need it. Clinical audit is a useful tool to monitor and improve practice against agreed guidelines looking at both the transfusion process and appropriateness of transfusion. In order for audit to be successful, the cycle must be completed to include the following:

♦ Change implemented where necessary.
♦ Results and educational messages must be disseminated and discussed.
♦ Analysis of corrective actions are required to improve practice.
♦ Analysis of change in practice.
♦ Provision of resources required to implement change.

The blood bank and the transfusion practitioners can provide support for audit and monitoring:

♦ Internal laboratory audits to assess compliance with laboratory process.
♦ Retrospective and/or prospective audit of appropriateness of transfusion.
♦ Audit of indications for transfusion.
♦ Administration of blood components.
♦ Regular audits of the Maximum Surgical Blood Order Schedule (MSBOS). The blood bank needs to be able to provide blood components for both routine and emergency procedures. Most laboratories will provide a MSBOS, which lists the number of units routinely provided for each surgical procedure. It is important the MSBOS is reviewed on a regular basis to allow:

• Reduction in workload of unnecessary crossmatching.
• Improved stock management and wastage.
• The tariff to be agreed by all parties.
• For change in clinical practice that may lead to changes in blood support needed.
• The monitoring of practice.

The SHOT scheme can provide information which allows targeting of problem areas, particularly in the transfusion process.

Role in the support of autologous service

The role of the hospital blood bank in support of any autologous service is integral to the success of the service. Each hospital will need to determine which system(s) or process will best suit their needs:

♦ Pre-deposit.
♦ Intra-operative cell salvage.
♦ Postoperative drainage and re-infusion

The hospital blood bank has a role to play in the development and implementation of training programmes and competency assessments that are needed to underpin a successful autologous service. They can also support the quality control and data collection aspects of an autologous service.

Future activities

The blood bank has a definite role to play in:

♦ Evaluating and introducing more secure means of patient identification.
♦ Blood fridge and bedside tracking of blood component movements.
♦ Appropriate ordering and use of blood components as indicated by national guidelines or local variations thereof.
♦ Development of transfusion avoidance strategies.
♦ Recording the transfusion process from "vein-to-vein".
♦ Recognition of transfusion reactions apart from Acute Transfusion Reaction (ATR) and Delayed Transfusion Reaction (DTR).

Key Summary

◆   Blood transfusion is an integral part of clinical practice.

◆   Communication, with all persons involved in the transfusion process, is an integral part of blood transfusion.

◆   It is important that the blood bank facilitates transfusion support for patients which is timely, safe and clinically appropriate.

◆   Blood is a valuable and increasingly scarce resource. Transfusion avoidance strategies are an important part of clinical practice and are to be implemented wherever possible.

◆   The facilitation of audit, education, critical incident reporting and corrective action strategies is an important area where blood banks need to be involved.

References

1.   NHS Executive. Better Blood Transfusion. Department of Health, London, 1998 (Health Service Circular 1998/224).
2.   NHS Executive. Better Blood Transfusion: Appropriate Use of Blood. Department of Health, London, 2002 (Health Service Circular 2002/009).
3.   EC Directive 2002/98/EC, OJC 33.8.2003: 30-80.

Chapter 7

Acute Normovolaemic Haemodilution

Richard J Telford BSc (Hons) MB BS FRCA
Consultant Anaesthetist
Jonathan M Hall B Med Sci (Hons) BM BS MRCP FRCA
Specialist Registrar
Royal Devon and Exeter Hospital, Exeter, UK

"There is little level one evidence that ANH alone spares significant quantities of allogeneic blood."

Introduction

Since its introduction in the 1970s[1] acute normovolaemic haemodilution (ANH) has been advocated as a technique to reduce the exposure of patients to homologous blood.

Blood conservation strategies have become increasingly important in the 21st century as the safety of homologous blood transfusions has been questioned. Transmitted viral infections have become an increasing public and professional concern.

In addition, blood is a commodity which is in short supply. Each year in the UK, demand for blood increases by 2-3%, reflecting our ageing population and the increased complexity of medical and surgical procedures requiring transfusion. It has been predicted that there may be a shortfall of red cells soon if present patterns of blood donation continue.

Problems with the supply of blood have been exacerbated in the UK in 2004 by the exclusion from the donor pool of those who have received a blood transfusion since 1980. This is an attempt to further minimise the theoretical risk of the transmission of variant Creutzfeldt-Jakob disease (vCJD) by homologous blood transfusion.

One method of blood conservation is acute normovolaemic haemodilution which involves the immediate pre-operative collection of whole blood from the patient with simultaneous infusion of crystalloid or colloid to maintain normovolaemia. ANH can be performed immediately before or after the onset of anaesthesia. Blood is withdrawn into citrated blood bags, which may be stored at room temperature for six hours. This may be prolonged to 12 hours with appropriate cooling.

ANH has several advantages over autologous blood donation:

♦ The blood procured by haemodilution requires no testing.
♦ The blood is fresh, containing functional platelets and clotting factors.
♦ The units are not removed from the operating theatre, so the possibility of an administrative error resulting in an ABO incompatible blood transfusion, is virtually eliminated.
♦ Bacterial contamination is less likely.
♦ Blood obtained by haemodilution does not require substantial investment of time by the patient as it is obtained at the time of surgery.

Indications

Current UK guidelines state that ANH should be considered when the potential surgical blood loss is likely to exceed 20% of the blood volume. Patients should have a pre-operative haemoglobin of more than 10g dl^{-1} and not have severe myocardial disease (leading to moderate to severe left ventricular impairment), unstable angina, severe aortic stenosis or critical left main stem coronary artery disease [2].

Compensatory mechanisms

The effect of reducing the haemoglobin concentration during ANH results in a decrease of the oxygen carrying capacity of arterial blood. In normal individuals an increase in cardiac output compensates for the decrease in arterial oxygen content, so that oxygen delivery is maintained.

The increase in cardiac output can be of such magnitude that during initial haemodilution augmented oxygen delivery may result.

Progressive haemodilution will ultimately decrease oxygen delivery. This does not initially compromise whole body oxygen consumption, as most organs are capable of increasing oxygen extraction. Redistribution of organ blood flow to the heart and brain is observed during extreme haemodilution.

The principal mechanisms of increased cardiac output are:-

♦ Reduced blood viscosity. Blood viscosity decreases exponentially with falling haemoglobin concentration. The steepest part of the curve occurs between haemoglobin concentrations of 15g dl^{-1} and 10g dl^{-1}. This increases venous return and reduces total peripheral resistance, increasing cardiac output.
♦ Increased sympathetic stimulation of the heart. This is related to the activation of aortic chemoreceptors and accounts for approximately one third of the increase in cardiac output.

Coronary physiology

In patients with normal coronary anatomy, there is a marked increase in coronary and myocardial blood flow with ANH. Active coronary vasodilatation and the effects of decreased blood viscosity, mean that myocardial oxygen delivery is well-maintained. It is the subendocardium that is most vulnerable to the effects of impaired oxygen delivery, particularly in the face of high metabolic demands.

Patients with coronary artery stenoses tolerate haemodilution less well; abnormalities of systolic and diastolic function may result. Coronary stenoses may limit the heart's ability to increase cardiac output during progressive haemodilution by decreasing the "recruitable" functional reserves of the left ventricle.

Calculating the volume of blood to be withdrawn

Calculation of the volume of blood to be withdrawn is done using the simplified formula published by Gross [3].

$$\text{Volume of blood to be removed} = \text{EBV (70ml kg}^{-1}) \times \frac{(H_i - H_f)}{H_{av}}$$

Where:
EBV = Estimated Blood Volume
H_i = Initial Haematocrit
H_f = Final Haematocrit
H_{av} = Average of H_i and H_f

The haemoglobin concentration is most easily measured by a near patient testing device such as the Hemocue®. The haematocrit is obtained by multiplying the haemoglobin concentration by three.

Technique of pre-operative haemodilution

♦ The calculated volume of blood is withdrawn from a venous or arterial line connected to a three-way stopcock into citrated collection bags.
♦ Haemodilution kits that contain a Y type Luer locking adapter simplify the procedure and improve sterility (Figure 1).
♦ Use of a spring balance allows the volume of blood withdrawn to be measured.
♦ 450-500ml of blood is withdrawn into each bag which is gently agitated during the collection process until the target haematocrit is reached.

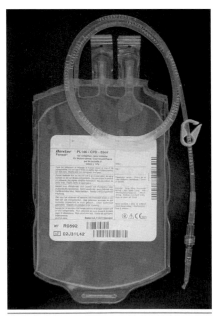

Figure 1. Haemodilution kit (courtesy of Baxter Ltd.).

♦ The bags containing the autologous blood are labelled, numbered sequentially and stored at room temperature to maintain platelet function.

♦ Occasionally, the collection process may be prolonged during the initial phase of surgery, but it must be finished before significant surgical blood loss occurs.

♦ Since the first unit of autologous blood obtained is richest in red cells, platelets and clotting factors, it should be retransfused last, ideally at the end of surgery when surgical haemostasis has been obtained.

♦ Any autologous blood remaining after surgery may be stored at 4°C for up to 12 hours. Cooling however, affects platelet function.

Choice of replacement fluid

Euvolaemic patients maintain cardiac output and oxygen delivery to the tissues. Blood should therefore be replaced with a suitable substitute. Ideally, this substitute should have a similar colloid osmotic pressure to plasma.

If synthetic colloids are used a 1:1 replacement ratio is reasonable. The modified fluid gelatins (Gelofusine®, Hacmaccel®) have a short (2-3 hour) intravascular half-life due to their low average molecular weight. The hydroxyethyl starches (HES) are a better choice as replacement fluid due to their longer intravascular half-life (12-18 hours).

Crystalloids can also be used. They have a short intravascular half-life and infusion of large volumes aggravate tissue oedema. Normal saline and Hartmann's solution equilibrate between the intravascular and the interstitial space. If they are chosen to maintain normovolaemia, a 3:1 replacement ratio needs to be used (data from the recent SAFE study suggest a lower ratio [1:1.5] may be adequate).

Human albumin solutions are not used because of the issues surrounding variant Creutzfeldt-Jakob disease, along with cost and efficacy.

Efficacy

ANH is employed alongside other blood conservation measures to minimise the exposure of patients to homologous blood. Mathematical modelling has suggested that severe haemodilution (pre-operative haemoglobin less than 20%) accompanied by substantial blood loss would be required before the red cell volume saved becomes clinically important [4].

Spahnl [5] has demonstrated that ANH to a haemoglobin concentration of 8.8+/-0.3g dl^{-1} was well tolerated in 20 patients older than 65 years. He also experienced no problems when haemodiluting 60 patients with coronary disease receiving ß-blockers to a haemoglobin concentration of 9.9+/-0.2g dl^{-1} [6]. However, Carvalho [7] reported a case of life-threatening myocardial ischaemia in a patient undergoing ANH prior to elective abdominal aortic aneurysm repair.

Consensus conferences in Edinburgh [8,9] noted that there was still no evidence that ANH was effective, concluding that randomised controlled trials were required before ANH could be recommended.

The quality of published studies on ANH is still not good enough to make any firm conclusions about its efficacy and the numbers studied are so small that the doubts about the safety of the technique remain unresolved.

Transfusion triggers

The haemoglobin concentration at which to transfuse patients is variable and must be decided on an individual patient basis. There is no evidence that a liberal transfusion policy improves outcome and some evidence that a restrictive transfusion strategy may improve outcome [10].

Clinical guidelines suggest that transfusion is rarely indicated if the haemoglobin is greater than 10g dl^{-1} and usually indicated if the haemoglobin is less than 6g dl^{-1} in clinically stable patients not at risk of coronary disease [11]. Patients with coronary artery disease may require a higher transfusion trigger.

Future developments

Haemoglobin-based oxygen carriers (HBOC) have been under investigation for many years. Modification of the free haemoglobin tetramer by cross-linking and polymerization, has produced solutions with intravascular half-lives of around 24 hours with P_{50}s in the physiological range. It is possible in the near future that HBOCs will be used to maintain normovolaemia during ANH. It has been suggested that they may provide better haemodynamic stability and increase tissue oxygen tension when compared to hydroxyethyl starch.

Erythropoietin acts by stimulating erythropoiesis. It has been used to increase the efficacy of acute normovolaemic haemodilution by raising the pre-operative haemoglobin. This permits a greater volume of blood to be removed when ANH is performed. It has been used in Jehovah's Witnesses to permit major elective surgery (eg. liver transplantation) without exposure to allogeneic blood. It remains, however, an expensive method of minimising allogeneic blood transfusions [12].

There is little level one evidence to suggest that ANH alone spares significant quantities of allogeneic blood. Its use should be considered in conjunction with other blood conservation techniques as part of an integrated approach to minimise the exposure of patients to homologous blood.

Key Summary

◆ Acute normovolaemic haemodilution (ANH) involves the immediate pre-operative collection of whole blood from the patient with simultaneous infusion of crystalloid or colloid to maintain normovolaemia.

◆ It provides fresh blood, containing functional platelets and clotting factors.

◆ Current UK guidelines state that ANH should be considered when the potential surgical blood loss is likely to exceed 20% of the blood volume.

◆ There is very little (level one) evidence that it saves significant quantities of homologous blood.

◆ ANH should be used in conjunction with other methods of blood conservation to minimize the exposure of patients to homologous blood.

References

1.   Mesmer K. Haemodilution. *Surg Clin North Am* 1975; 55: 659.
2.   Napier JA, Bruce M, Chapman, *et al*. Guidelines for autologous transfusion II. Perioperative haemodilution and cell salvage. *Br J Anaes* 1997; 78: 768 - 771.
3.   Gross JB. Estimating allowable blood loss: corrected for dilution. *Anesthesiology* 1983; 58: 277-280.
4.   Brecher ME, Rosenfeld M. Mathematical and computer modelling of acute normovolaemic haemodilution. *Transfusion* 1994; 34: 176 - 179.
5.   Spahn DR, *et al*. Hemodilution tolerance in elderly patients without known cardiac disease. *Anesth Analg* 1996; 82: 681-686.
6.   Spahn DR, Schmid ER, Seifert B, Pasch T. Hemodilution tolerance in patients with coronary artery disease who are receiving chronic beta-adrenergic blocker therapy. *Anesth Analg* 1996; 82: 687-694.
7.   Carvalho B, Ridler BM, Thompson JF, Telford RJ. Myocardial ischaemia precipitated by acute normovolaemic haemodilution. *Transfus Med* 2003; 13: 165-168.
8.   Thomas MJ. Royal College of Physicians of Edinburgh Consensus Conference on autologous transfusion: final consensus statement. *Transfus Sci* 1996; 17: 329-330.

9. Allain JP, Akehurst RL, Hunter JM. Royal College of Physicians of Edinburgh. Autologous transfusion, 3 years on: What is new? What has happened? *Transfusion* 1999; 39: 910-911.

10. Hebert PC, Wells G, *et al.* A multicenter, randomized, controlled clinical trial of transfusion requirements in critical care. Transfusion Requirements in Critical Care Investigators, Canadian Critical Care Trials Group. *N Engl J Med* 1999; 340: 409-417.

11. Practice Guidelines for blood component therapy: A report by the American Society of Anesthesiologists Task Force on Blood Component Therapy. *Anesthesiology* 1996; 84: 732-747.

12. Goodnough LT, Monk TG, Andriole GL. Current concepts: erythropoietin therapy. *N Engl J Med* 1997; 336: 933-938.

Chapter 8

Intra-operative Cell Salvage

John F Thompson MS FRCSEd FRCS

Consultant Surgeon, Royal Devon and Exeter Hospital, Exeter, UK

"Most hospitals running an ICS service are quite happy with its cost savings, quality improvement and governance issues, and all patients receiving their own blood are grateful for the opportunity."

Introduction

Whatever strategies are used to minimise a surgical patient's exposure to allogeneic blood, the final outcome depends on the amount of blood lost during the operation, both on the swabs and in suction. If this blood can be retrieved and re-infused safely to restore the circulating haematocrit above the "trigger" level which otherwise would have led to a transfusion, the principle of cell salvage is proven. Consensus conferences, Government directives and national guidelines have endorsed Intra-operative Cell Salvage (ICS) as an effective strategy which should be widely available [1,2,3]. This chapter describes the different devices and how a service can be established.

Efficacy of ICS

Level one evidence of the efficacy of ICS is sparse but convincing, especially in vascular, cardiac and orthopaedic surgery [4,5]. The problem is that of the constantly changing environment where ICS is used. Enthusiasts generally work in a hospital where there is an active blood conservation programme and where surgeons are careful not to lose blood. However, all surgeons come across difficult cases where unexpected blood loss can occur. The strength of ICS is that as blood loss rises, efficiency improves also. The blood that is lost following a technical incident is usually clean and free-flowing - perfect for ICS, which is the "surgeon's safety net".

Negative studies come from units where, for example, the ICS service is provided commercially. The company's operator has to attend the surgery, so disposables are opened as a matter of routine, whether needed or not.

Technical improvements in surgery emerge all the time. For example, in cardiac surgery, ICS is now seldom actually used for first-time coronary artery bypass grafting, but is very efficient for valve replacement or re-do cases. However, it is useful to always have the machine on standby for unexpected incidents, such as a tie coming off an aorto-coronary graft, so that the pump blood can be concentrated and re-infused.

Indications change over time and usually out-pace the literature. Most hospitals running an ICS service are quite happy with its cost savings, quality improvement and governance issues, and all patients receiving their own blood are grateful for the opportunity.

Methods

ICS is divided into two main approaches:

♦ Washed systems (centrifugal, rotary and filtration).
♦ Unwashed systems.

Washed systems

Blood is anticoagulated at the point of collection - at the sucker tip - with either heparin (30,000iu/l) or citrate. Citrate is available in pre-prepared litre bags. Shed blood is collected in a suitable reservoir. When sufficient

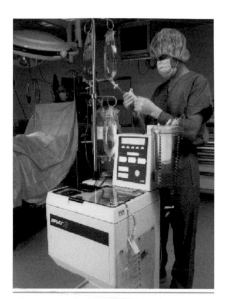

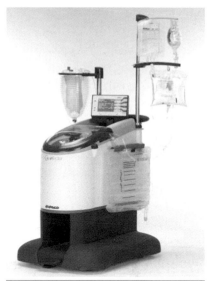

Figure 1. Cobe BRAT 2 (courtesy of Cobe Cardiovascular Inc.).

Figure 2. Sorin Electa (courtesy of Sorin Biomedica UK Ltd).

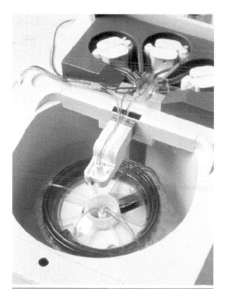

Figure 3. The CATS device showing the rotor system for cell separation.

has been collected the processing disposables are loaded which enable the blood to be either spun in a centrifuge (Haemonetics, COBE [Figure 1], Sorin [Figure 2], Electromedics) or passed through a rotor device (Fresenius CATS [Figure 3]). The blood is then washed by passing saline through it and pumped into a re-infusion bag. The system can be continuous, which is acceptable for Jehovah's Witness patients.

Washout efficiency is typically 95-98% for most plasma phase contaminants and 75-80% of the blood lost can be

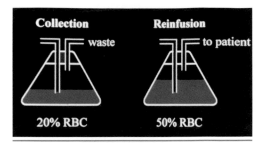

Figure 4. Centrifugal cell washers act as a red cell trap which increases the haematocrit of the re-infusate.

returned. The centrifuge traps red cells, increasing the haematocrit of the re-infusate to 60-70% (Figure 4) [6]. Swabs laden with blood can be washed out in bowls of saline which can be processed.

Unwashed systems

Blood is collected in a passive reservoir via a short suction tube (Figure 5). Shear stress at the sucker tip is a strong stimulus for coagulation so the patient must be anticoagulated with heparin 2mg/kg. Non-washed ICS is only suitable for vascular or cardiac surgery and only during the heparinised phase. If protamine sulphate is used to reverse heparin (there is evidence that this will increase bleeding) the reservoir will clot. In some cases of ruptured aneurysm the system can be used because of the coagulopathy associated with the condition.

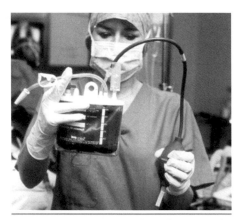

Figure 5. An example of a simple reservoir device; excess air is being bled out of the container to avoid the risk of air embolus on re-infusion.

Safety

It is difficult to find cases where ICS has led to adverse events, unless there has been a technical failure or the machine has been used incorrectly. Papers dealing with potential problems have disappeared from the literature. In summary:

♦ Platelets are activated during salvage and consumed by normal intra-operative clotting. The relatively few platelets salvaged play no effective part in coagulation. Platelet transfusion may be required to supplement high volume ICS (at least an exchange transfusion).

♦ Fibrinolysis is a prominent biochemical feature of ICS because the salvaged blood has usually already undergone clotting and lysis within the cavity it has been salvaged from. High D-Dimer levels are the norm, but do not reflect on-going Disseminated Intravascular Coagulation (DIC). D-Dimer is largely removed by washing but even if it is not, there is no evidence that its re-infusion is harmful.

♦ Leukocytes, complement and kinins are activated by both surgery and salvage but a systemic inflammatory response has not been reported, even using non-washed systems. Acute inflammatory mediators are removed by cell washing; the only adverse papers in the literature involved non-heparinised dogs with repeated cycling of blood through a centrifuge. Kinin activation may actually boost the immunity of the recipient (see Chapter 12) [7].

♦ Anticoagulant overdose is associated with filtration devices (Haemocell) because the filters rapidly block in clinical practice so that the heparin passes straight through to the recipient.

♦ Air embolus is no longer a problem with modern equipment when it is used correctly.

♦ Amniotic fluid contamination is avoided by a combination of cell washing and use of a leucocyte filter, such as the LeukoGuard® RS filter (Pall Medical) [8].

There are several "quirks" in ICS practice; for example antibiotics and some anaesthetics are removed, so supplemental doses may be required. Betadine and other washouts should be avoided as should topical haemostats. A double wash should be used to remove fat in orthopaedic surgery.

The areas of controversy in ICS are its use in sepsis and malignancy.

ICS in sepsis

ICS is useful and safe in trauma surgery so long as blood volume is maintained and broad spectrum antibiotics are given; good experimental and clinical literature supports this. In surgery where there may be contamination by bowel contents (such as cystectomy with ileal loop diversion), ICS is safe provided antibiotics are given and the clinician feels that the benefits of ICS outweigh the implications of homologous blood transfusion. ICS is contraindicated in most cases of septic revision arthroplasty for obvious reasons.

ICS in malignancy

This is a most interesting area. All authorities agree that there is sufficient evidence to reduce homologous blood transfusion in cancer surgery to reduce immune suppression, decrease peri-operative infections (wound, chest, urine) and possibly improve cancer-free survival. The two schools of thought are based on the following underlying principles:

◆ Viable cancer cells can be salvaged, washed by ICS devices and grown in nude mice. Nucleated cells are rendered sterile by 50Gy irradiation. Salvaged blood should always be irradiated before re-infusion, and filtered to remove residual cells [9]. Critics of this policy state that it is expensive, unnecessary and takes too long to be useful in most hospitals.

◆ Clinical studies (in urology, sarcoma surgery and other malignancies), involving many hundreds of patients, have failed to demonstrate the dissemination of blood-borne metastases by re-infusion of ICS blood from the tumour bed, despite the demonstration of circulating cancer cells [10]. Critics state that any risk of re-infusing even a single viable cell is unacceptable and that the studies to-date lack the statistical power to demonstrate the excess risk.

Those interested in using ICS will find cancer surgery one of the best indications for the technique. The advantages must be set against the potential risks, discussed amongst the clinicians involved, and outlined fully to the individual patient about to undergo surgery.

Table 1. Operations performed that potentially warrant a need for ICS.

Vascular surgery	**Urology**
Elective aortic aneurysm	Cystectomy
Thoraco-abdominal reconstruction	Radical prostatectomy
Emergency aortic surgery	Radical nephrectomy
	Orthotopic bladder reconstruction
Cardiac surgery	**Obstetrics and Gynaecology**
Valve replacement	Radical pelvic surgery
Aortic arch surgery	Ectopic pregnancy
Redo surgery	Difficult Caesarean section
Paediatrics	
Orthopaedics	
Primary hip arthroplasty (standby)	
Revision arthroplasty (aseptic)	
Spinal instrumentation	
Trauma	
(Resection for malignancy)	

Setting up a cell salvage service

As with all new developments, the first stage is to establish a business case, which follows a clinical case of need. All hospitals must have a transfusion committee where comparative audit data are considered. ICS will be an advantage if the hospital regularly performs those operations listed in Table 1.

The list in Table 1 is not exhaustive; all procedures involving the following should be considered for ICS:

- Blood loss >700-800ml.
- Routine transfusion of approximately 50% of cases.
- Reasonable rate of blood loss.
- Suitable site for salvage of blood.
- No contraindications to ICS.

Problems in establishing an ICS service

The potential barriers to the establishment of a service have been investigated by the clinical audit department of the National Blood Service, which found the following problems [11]:

♦ Lack of awareness of the role of autologous transfusion as a whole in modern clinical practice.
♦ Lack of awareness of the indications for ICS.
♦ Logistic difficulties.
♦ Financial barriers.
♦ Training operatives.
♦ Inertia/unwillingness to change.

The essential component in all successful hospitals is a lead clinician willing to develop the service, working alongside a Transfusion Practitioner. The impetus for change should be presented to the Hospital Risk Management Team and Executive Board, and the case should include:

♦ The need to comply with Directives relating to the introduction of improved blood management (in the UK this is part of a hospital's accreditation and clinical negligence assessment).
♦ Cell salvage as a component of that strategy.
♦ Governance issues relating to the avoidable exposure of patients to allogeneic blood.
♦ A local strategy to deal with problems with the supply of donor blood (in the UK there are national plans which will restrict non-essential surgery should there be a crisis).

Education

Education sessions should be held to engage stakeholders and especially those who will be running and using the ICS service. In our experience anaesthetists and theatre staff are the most important; presentations at departmental audit meetings and demonstrations of the available equipment are well-received.

Choice of device

The next stage is to decide on the device to be used. This is a matter of personal choice and economics. We evaluated several machines, compiled a check list and had a meeting where the relative merits were discussed from the perspective of the operator, surgeon, anaesthetist and the type of procedure. For example, the COBE BRAT II is suited to rapid re-infusion of large volumes in cardiac surgery, whereas the CATS or the Electa devices are perfect for paediatric orthopaedic surgery.

Finance

Finance departments will have little objection to ICS [12]. Several studies have shown it to be either cost neutral or negative; the main consideration is that the appropriate budgetary transfer is essential. Many hospitals have failed to implement ICS due to internecine disputes between departments, and in the author's view the funding should be "top-sliced".

ICS machines may be purchased outright or lease-purchased with a service contract. There are many possible combinations and most companies are willing to negotiate, depending on the number of disposables to be used.

Training

Training is a local issue. The most effective operatives are anaesthetic staff, both medical and technical, as they are familiar with a clinical/technical interface and are present throughout the ICS process. It is not necessary for technical staff to have an exhaustive knowledge of haematology and transfusion medicine, but they do need to be properly trained in the safe operation of the machine and its contraindications (in much the same way as they relate to anaesthetic machines). It is the doctor who has overall responsibility for the re-infusion of blood and if there are any queries, the responsible clinician should arbitrate.

PERI-OPERATIVE AUTOLOGOUS BLOOD SALVAGE RECORD	PATIENT IDENTIFICATION		
Date / /	Location Theatre: Recovery: ICU: Unit:		
Operator (Please print)	Operator Signature		
Auto-Transfusion Machine	Haemodilution Volume		
Volume Processed	Disposables	Serial No.	Expiry Date
Units (volume) given			
	Reinfusion bag		
	Collection Reservoir		
	Bowl Assembly		
	Suction Assembly		
Other Transfused Units	Aspiration Set		
RBC PLTS	Saline (09%)		
FFP CRYO	Anticoagulant		
	Pre-op Lab Results Hb _____ APTR _____ INR _____		
Anticoagulant Amount: Heparin _____ Citrate _____			
Comments: To ICU/Ward Staff	**PROCEDURE:** .... Emergency / Urgent / Elective		
	Epidural YES / NO		
	Surgeon:		
	Anaesthetist:		
Office use only:-			
24 hour postoperative Hb		Date of discharge from Hospital:	
One week postoperative Hb Postoperative blood bank transfusion Postoperative infection		Comments:	

Figure 3. Royal Devon and Exeter hospital's vascular service proforma recording the use of peri-operative autologous blood salvage.

Equipment manufacturers are very willing to set up training and certification sessions for staff (we hold these at weekends). A competency certificate for ICS is a useful addition to a technician's C.V. and an important part of a junior anaesthetist's training. Following a theoretical course, operators should make every effort to attend clinical cases to maintain their familiarity with the equipment. Many develop a great pride in providing this important service which can save lives.

Providing an ICS service out of hours is vital, as many trauma cases and ruptured aneurysms are admitted after hours. It makes sense to pay staff a call-out fee per case, which is economically viable when compared to the cost of blood saved.

Audit and quality control

Each case involving the use of ICS should be recorded prospectively to comply with traceability regulations regarding disposables and the machine used. There are several suitable proformas available (Royal Devon and Exeter hospital's proforma is shown in Figure 3). It is helpful to record cases on a computerised database for audit and research purposes and even more so if the database interfaces with that of the blood bank. Cases where the "collect only" software are used should be recorded. Adverse events should be reported to the Serious Hazards of Transfuion (SHOT) reporting system via the Hospital Transfusion Committee (HTC) as there is no separate recording mechanism for autologous blood transfusion.

Quality control samples should be sent at regular intervals. We record haematocrit, microbiological cultures and heparin levels (recently abandoned in favour of citrate) every month with results copied to the machine operator and responsible clinician.

Consent

At present, there is no special requirement for patients to give consent for blood transfusion. The potential use of ICS is however, discussed with patients under our care and recorded in the case-notes.

A Manual for Blood Conservation

> # Key Summary
>
> ◆ ICS is a quality issue in modern hospital practice.
> ◆ ICS should be available in cardiac, vascular and orthopaedic theatres.
> ◆ ICS should be considered for oncological surgery.
> ◆ A responsible clinician should oversee the service.
> ◆ The HTC should monitor outcomes and audit ICS.
> ◆ Adverse events should be reported to SHOT.

References

1. Autologous transfusion - 3 years on: what is new? What has happened? *Transfus Med* 1999; 9: 258-6.
2. NHS Executive. Better Blood Transfusion: Appropriate Use of Blood. Department of Health, London, 2002 (Health Service Circular 2002/009).
3. Peri-operative Blood Transfusion for Elective Surgery. http://www.sign.ac.uk.
4. Thompson JF, Chant ADB, Webster JHH. Prospective randomised evaluation of a new cell saving device in elective aortic reconstruction. *Eur J Vasc Surg* 1990; 4: 507-12.
5. Huet C, Salmi LR, Fergusson D, Koopman Van-Gemert AW, Rubens F, Laupacis A. A meta-analysis of cell-salvage to minimise perioperative blood transfusion in cardiac and orthopaedic surgery. International Study of Perioperative Transfusion Investigators (ISPOT) *Anesth Analg* 1999; 89: 861-9.
6. Ridler BMF, Thompson JF. The qualities of blood reinfused during cell salvage. *TATM* 2003; 5: 466-471.
7. Gharehbaghian A, Haquek KMG,Truman C, Evans R, Morse R, Newman J, Bannister G, Rogers C, Bradley B. Effect of autologous salvaged blood on postoperative natural killer cell precursor frequency. *Lancet* 2004; 363: 1025-3.
8. Waters JH, Biscotti C, Potter PS, Phillipson E. Amniotic fluid removal during cell salvage in the Caesarean section patient. *Anesthesiology* 2000; 92: 1531-6.
9. Hansen E, Bechmann V, Altmeppen J. Intraoperative blood salvage in oncologic surgery. Answers to current questions. *Infus Therap Transfus Med* 2002; 29: 138-41.
10. Davis M, Sofer M, Gomez-Marin O, Bruck D, Soloway MS. The use of the cell saver during radical retropubic prostatectomy: does it influence recurrence? *BJU Int* 2003; 91: 474-6.
11. James V, Lamb J. The contribution of a blood establishment to the increased use of intraoperative cell salvage in hospitals: a pilot study from the national blood service, England. *TATM* 2003; 5: 484-8.
12. Morgan C, Cooper M. Cell Salvage in Cardiothoracic Surgery - Cost issues. *TATM* 2003: 5: 461-5.

Chapter 9

Surgical Methods to Minimise Blood Loss

John V Taylor MB ChB, FRCS (Ed)
Specialist Registrar, Vascular Surgery
Francesco Torella MD FRCS (Gen)
Consultant Vascular Surgeon, Honorary Senior Lecturer in Surgery
University Hospital Aintree, Liverpool, UK

"Individual surgical technique is highly variable and probably remains the most relevant factor."

Introduction

Operative intervention is, by its very nature, destructive and will result in damage to blood vessels and thus loss of blood. The aim of surgical dissection is to obtain a rapid and safe incision of tissues without damage to surrounding structures and with minimal blood loss. Individual surgical technique is highly variable and probably remains the most relevant factor in achieving this goal. In many circumstances, a good technique, developing avascular tissue planes with pre-emptive ligation of sizable blood vessels, ensures a bloodless field. Not uncommonly however, this cannot be achieved because of pathological changes in the tissues, or because surgery is performed on highly vascular structures.

Advances in technology have allowed the development of specific techniques and tools to aid the surgeon with haemostasis (and blood conservation in general) in the most diverse of circumstances. This chapter describes the role of such methods in modern surgical practice.

General measures

There are a number of simple expedients to aid blood conservation; although these can be employed without resorting to expensive equipment,

Table 1. General measures to aid blood conservation.

Meticulous dissection
Develop avascular planes
Stop all small bleeders as encountered
Reduction of regional vascular pressure
Appropriate patient position
Blood inflow control
Limb exsanguination
Prevention of hypothermia
Heating blankets
Avoid unnecessary evisceration
Avoid cold washout solutions and fluid spillage onto porous drapes
Optimal use of cell salvage

they may be often overlooked (Table 1). Due to their simplicity, they should be considered in every procedure where significant blood loss is a possibility.

Surgical dissection

As a general rule, bleeding should be stopped as soon as it is encountered during dissection. Although many small vessels will eventually seal spontaneously after division, ignoring these bleeding points during extensive surgery may lead to significant blood loss, which is difficult to both quantify and control.

Control of regional vascular pressure

The volume of blood lost from a damaged vessel depends on the capacity of the vessel, the size of the tear, haemostatic mechanisms such as vasospasm and blood clotting, and blood pressure. The latter can be controlled to a degree by simple measures, such as modifying the position

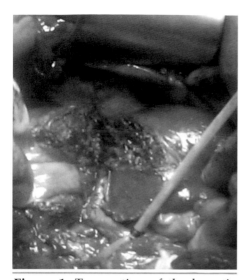

Figure 1. Transection of the hepatic parenchyma during extended right hepatectomy. A tourniquet snug around the hepatic hilum and a low central venous pressure ensure a bloodless field. The hepatic tissue is divided by CUSA (see page 96) and small vessels are sealed by the argon beam coagulator.

of the patient. Elevating the operating field above the heart produces a drop in the regional arterial and venous pressure. The effect on the arterial pressure is small, but the regional venous circulation can be almost emptied by suitable positioning. This is commonly used in lower limb venous surgery (head down) and in head and neck surgery (head up). The same result is achieved in spinal surgery by supporting the patient, avoiding any contact between the abdomen and the operating table, thus reducing back-pressure from the caval circulation to the vertebral veins [1].

When bloodless dissection is desirable, the surgeon may elect to interrupt blood inflow to the operated organ. This is done during hepatic resections by clamping the hepatic artery and the portal vein at the hilum of the liver during division of the parenchyma, while lowering central venous pressure to reduce venous back-bleeding from the hepatic venous circulation (Figure 1) [2]. Similarly, blood loss may be reduced during extensive pelvic surgery by clamping the infrarenal aorta [3].

Complete elimination of bleeding is possible in some orthopaedic, plastic or vascular procedures on limbs, as anaesthetised skin, muscle and bone tolerate ischaemia well. A bloodless field can be maintained with a high-pressure tourniquet, after exsanguination of the limb (Figure 2). This technique, often used during knee surgery, offers the additional advantage that postoperative cell salvage can be used to its full potential, because blood loss is limited to the postoperative period.

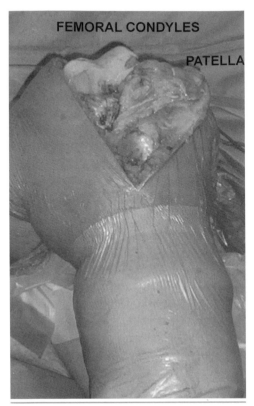

FEMORAL CONDYLES

PATELLA

Figure 2. Total knee replacement: exsanguination and a proximal tourniquet ensure a bloodless operative field.

Maintenance of normothermia

This is essential to preserve platelet function and hence haemostasis [4]. Temperature monitoring and prevention of hypothermia are largely the responsibility of the anaesthetist, but the surgical team can contribute by minimising temperature losses from the operative field. This can be achieved by measures, such as the avoidance of unnecessary evisceration of bowel during abdominal procedures, the use of warm, rather than cold, washout solutions and the prevention of fluid spillage through drapes. Disposable impermeable drapes decrease evaporative loss and help to maintain normothermia.

Optimal use of cell salvage

Cell salvage is an established blood conservation technique that allows re-infusion of a proportion of the red cells lost to suction. A variable amount of blood, however, is removed from the operative field by swabs and normally not recycled but these swabs can be washed in isotonic solution and the resultant fluid processed. This increases the amount of salvaged blood by approximately one third during aortic aneurysm repair, with a similar red cell yield to suctioned blood [5]. The proportion of blood saved may be higher in other operations where swabs are used in preference to suction.

Surgical access

Many major surgical procedures require long incisions and extensive dissection to expose and treat the target pathology. The morbidity associated with this type of surgery has driven surgeons to explore minimally invasive techniques. These are generally based on endoscopy (including laparoscopy and thoracoscopy) or image guidance (radiology, ultrasound), which, in some cases, can be performed entirely percutaneously (for example, ablation of hepatic tumours). An additional benefit of these approaches is reduced blood loss. This is a function of a combination of factors, including smaller incisions, more localised dissection, the use of magnifying imaging systems and "haemostatic" instruments. Examples of minimally invasive surgical procedures with smaller blood losses than their conventional counterparts are endovascular repair of abdominal aortic aneurysms [6] and laparoscopic colonic resections [7].

"Traditional" operations will remain in widespread use for some time, until the new techniques are properly evaluated, specialised equipment becomes available and a sufficient number of surgeons are trained to perform them.

Cardiac surgery constitutes a special case, due to the emergence of off-pump coronary artery bypass (OfCAB). Although not strictly minimally invasive, this technique results in better peri-operative platelet function than surgery on cardiopulmonary bypass [8] and has been shown, in a randomised trial, to reduce blood loss and transfusion requirements [9].

Surgical instruments

A variety of instruments are available that allow division or disruption of target tissue with simultaneous sealing of blood vessels (Table 2). The majority rely on the transfer of thermal energy, acting by a combination of protein denaturation and clot formation to form a surface coagulum. A potential drawback of these instruments is collateral damage to nearby tissue due to heat transmission, which limits their applicability because of these safety concerns. More recent developments include ultrasonic and water-jet dissectors, which, although expensive, generate a lesser degree of thermal energy.

Table 2. "Haemostatic" dissecting instruments.

	Mechanism of action	Disadvantages	Common applications
Monopolar diathermy	Heat transmission	Collateral thermal damage Interference with pacemakers Ignition of flammable fluid/gas	Most procedures
Bipolar diathermy	Heat transmission	Cannot "cut" tissues Ignition of flammable fluid/gas	Most procedures where precise dissection is required
Argon Beam Coagulator	Heat transmission	Collateral thermal damage Interference with pacemakers Ignition of flammable fluid/gas	Hepatobiliary surgery
Laser	Heat transmission	Collateral thermal damage Ignition of flammable fluid/gas Cost Eye injury	According to the type of laser
Ultrasound dissector	Mechanical disruption Some heat transmission	Cost	Surgery on solid organs
Water-jet dissector	Mechanical disruption	Cost	Surgery on solid organs

Diathermy

The passage of high frequency (>50 KHz) alternating current through the body is not harmful and does not stimulate muscular contraction. Surgical diathermy uses this current to deliver a localised thermal injury to target tissues. Modern diathermy was introduced to surgical practice by Harvey Cushing in 1926 and is now used in most surgical procedures.

Monopolar diathermy

Monopolar diathermy relies on the passage of current from a small electrode tip through the body to a large surface area return plate placed at a distant site. Heat is produced at the electrode tip, where the current is maximally concentrated, and results in tissue disruption and coagulation. The return plate dissipates the heat. For coagulation, the current is applied in bursts, to desiccate tissues; this in turn distorts blood vessels, denaturates plasma proteins and locally stimulates the clotting cascade. Monopolar diathermy can also be used to divide tissues, with sealing of small blood vessels. This effect is produced by the application of a continuous current, with a more extreme heating effect, turning intracellular water to steam and vaporising cells. A "blend" setting is now available in most diathermy machines to achieve a combination of cutting and coagulation.

In conventional monopolar diathermy, the current is delivered to the tissues by metal forceps tips or a blade. The Argon Beam Coagulator uses a stream of argon gas emitted from a hand-held electrode to deliver the current to the tissues. This device is particularly useful in the division and haemostasis of solid organs, such as the liver, as the argon stream has a larger contact area compared to a standard monopolar electrode. The flow of argon also helps to disperse oozing blood and cellular debris from the target area, resulting in more effective haemostatis.

Bipolar diathermy

Bipolar diathermy relies on the current travelling between two closely applied electrodes, usually forceps tips or scissor blades. Heat is thus only generated between the two electrodes, leading to a more localised, safer action than monopolar diathermy. Generally speaking, bipolar diathermy is useful in cases where the passage of a current through the body is undesirable, as in the presence of a cardiac pacemaker or other electrical implant, or when surgery is performed in close proximity to structures easily damaged by dispersed energy, such as nerves or thin-walled veins.

The Ligasure™ device is a particular type of bipolar diathermy in which the current travels between the jaws of a crushing clamp. It allows safe sealing of larger blood vessels than with standard bipolar diathermy and has been shown to reduce blood loss in several procedures such as haemorrhoidectomy [10], gastric surgery [11] and laparoscopic splenectomy [12].

Lasers

LASER (Light Amplification by Stimulated Emission of Radiation) uses a high-powered light source at a specific wavelength, reflected through a delivery system to produce a focused beam. When directed onto tissues, light is converted to thermal energy producing a diathermy-like effect. This is not only dependent on the power of the light beam, but also on the depth of penetration, which, in turn, is a function of the wavelength. Differences in physical properties of lasers thus determine their clinical application. Examples of lasers in common use are neodymium-yttrium-aluminium garnet (Nd-YAG), carbon dioxide (CO_2), argon and holmium-YAG.

Nd-YAG lasers

Nd-YAG lasers produce light at a wavelength of 1.06µm and penetrate to a depth of 3-5mm. They are frequently used to photocoagulate bleeding vessels endoscopically, such as in cases of acute gastrointestinal bleeding. The Nd-YAG laser is also useful in palliative endoluminal ablation of tumours in the gastrointestinal tract and in the treatment of benign prostatic hypertrophy.

CO_2 lasers

CO_2 lasers emit light at a wavelength of 10.6µm. As this light is rapidly absorbed by water the effect is limited to the most superficial layers only. CO_2 lasers are therefore mainly used in the destruction of surface tissues, as in the treatment of pre-cancerous lesions of the uterine cervix and skin.

Argon lasers

Argon lasers produce light at 0.49-0.51µm in the blue-green range, and are therefore absorbed by red pigments. Their main use lies in opthalmology to photocoagulate retinal lesions.

Holmium-YAG

Holmium-YAG lasers emit light at a wavelength of 2.1µm, which penetrates to a depth of 0.5-1mm. Their main field of application is in endourology, including lithotripsy, transurethral resection of bladder tumours or prostate, and pyeloplasty.

Cost is the principal drawback to the use of lasers and as most lasers for medical use are potentially dangerous (fire hazard, eye damage), appropriate safety measures must be implemented. A good example of lasers contributing to blood conservation is the endoscopic treatment of benign prostatic hypertrophy by holmium-YAG. This is largely a bloodless procedure, in contrast with diathermy resection, which leads to a variable but significant blood loss, occasionally requiring transfusion. After reviewing the available evidence, the National Institute for Clinical Excellence (UK) concluded that holmium-YAG prostatectomy is at least equivalent, and in some cases preferable, to standard transurethral prostatectomy, with the additional benefit of reduced blood loss [13].

Ultrasound and water-jet dissectors

These instruments have been largely developed for procedures requiring division of parenchymatous organs such as the liver. More traditional dissecting instruments are not precise enough to avoid damage to the many small blood vessels present in these vascular structures. The ultrasound-based harmonic scalpel consists of shears, or crushing jaws, vibrating at 55,500Hz. This energy disrupts cells but has little effect on collagen fibres. When applied to a solid organ, the parenchymal portion is divided, but hypocellular structures such as blood vessels, bile ducts and nerves, are left undamaged, with consequent reductions in blood loss and increased safety. The blood vessels, ducts or nerves encountered during dissection are then either preserved or ligated and divided under direct vision. Ultrasonic dissection is associated with modest heat generation, with temperatures between 50-100°C, in contrast to 150-1000°C produced by lasers and electrosurgical devices. A refinement of the ultrasonic dissector is the Cavitational Ultrasonic Surgical Aspirator (CUSA)(see Figure 1). This instrument incorporates an aspiration channel to remove fragments of disrupted tissue during dissection, allowing good visualisation of the operating field.

Water-jet dissectors are essentially based on the same principles of ultrasonic instruments, but the cells are disrupted by a high-pressure jet of saline solution. An aspirating channel ensures a clean operating field. Hypocellular, collagen-rich structures are preserved.

A number of studies support the use of ultrasound or water-jet dissectors to reduce blood loss [14-15]. Other authors however, have found little difference in comparison to traditional methods [16], confirming that the value of these expensive instruments cannot overshadow that of individual surgical technique. Surgeons should evaluate and where appropriate, incorporate these tools in their own strategy to optimise blood conservation.

Topical haemostatic agents

These are applied over a bleeding area to enhance clot formation. As a rule, they should only be used when blood loss cannot be controlled by more straightforward means such as the use of sutures, ligatures or diathermy. Topical haemostatic agents can be broadly divided in two groups:

♦ Haemostatic swabs.
♦ Fibrin sealants.

Haemostatic swabs

These provide a biodegradable scaffold upon which the patient's haemostatic mechanism can build a stable clot. A chemical or biological compound, such as calcium alginate, oxidised cellulose, thrombin or collagen promotes one or more steps of the clotting cascade. Such products are useful, inexpensive and widely used.

Fibrin sealants

These preparations provide an exogenous source of clot to stem bleeding independently of the patient's own haemostatic mechanism. They consist of separate sources of thrombin and fibrinogen. When mixed *in situ*, thrombin converts the fibrinogen to fibrin. Often an anti-fibrinolytic agent (usually aprotinin), factor XIII (a fibrin clot stabilizer) and calcium chloride, are added to the preparation [17]. Several manufacturers provide commercially available biodegradable preparations, with varying concentrations of the active compounds, but blood banks are a potential alternative source. These compounds are attractive because, theoretically, they can produce satisfactory haemostasis even in presence of coagulopathy.

Several studies of rather variable quality have evaluated the efficacy of topical haemostatic agents, often comparing one agent to another [18-19]. Interpretation of the evidence is hindered by a number of problems. These often include poor study design, surrogate outcome measures (time to complete haemostasis or suture line blood loss, rather than transfusion requirements) and narrow entry criteria, which prevent generalisation of results. Serious complications have been reported, particularly with oxidised cellulose sheets (probably the most commonly used haemostatic swab) causing foreign body reactions mimicking tumours or compressing nearby structures [20]. Despite these drawbacks, a recent Cochrane review cautiously supported the efficacy of fibrin sealants in reducing peri-operative blood loss and transfusion requirements [21].

Conclusions

Although individual surgical technique is the main determinant of peri-operative blood loss, an adequate blood conservation strategy must include a range of surgical adjuncts to reduce bleeding. Many of these, such as correct patient positioning, are simple and should be implemented in every case where blood loss is an issue. More expensive or advanced methods, such as the use of topical haemostatic agents and the use of "haemostatic" instruments, have been shown to reduce blood loss in certain circumstances. Although their effect on overall transfusion requirement is often uncertain, every surgeon should consider their use to optimise blood conservation.

Key Summary

◆ Surgical technique is the most important determinant of blood loss.

◆ Simple physical methods result in a significant reduction in blood loss.

◆ Minimally invasive surgery can contribute to blood conservation.

◆ Modern "haemostatic" surgical instruments can contribute to bloodless dissection, especially in operations on solid organs.

◆ Topical haemostatic agents, particularly fibrin sealants, are helpful when bleeding cannot be controlled by more straightforward means.

References

1.　Lee TC, Yang LC, Chen HJ. Effect of patient position and hypotensive anesthesia on inferior vena caval pressure. *Spine* 1998; 23: 941-7.

2.　Johnson M, Mannar R, Wu AW. Correlation between blood loss and inferior vena caval pressure during liver resection. *Br J Surg* 1998; 85: 188-90.

3.　Eisenkop SM, Spirtos NM, Lin WC, *et al*. Reduction of blood loss during extensive pelvic procedures by aortic clamping - a preliminary report. *Gynecol Oncol* 2003; 88: 80-4.

4.　Michelson AD, MacGregor H, Barnard MR, *et al*. Reversible inhibition of human platelet activation by hypothermia *in vivo* and *in vitro*. *Thromb Haemost* 1994; 71: 633-40.

5. Haynes SL, Bennett JR, Torella F, McCollum CN. Does swab washing improve red cell recovery in aortic surgery? *Vox Sang* 2004; 87(S3): 50.
6. Maher MM, McNamara AM, MacEneaney PM, *et al*.. Abdominal aortic aneurysms: elective endovascular repair versus conventional surgery - evaluation with evidence-based medicine techniques. *Radiology* 2003; 228: 647-58.
7. Lacy AM, Garcia-Valdecasas JC, Delgado S, *et al*. Laparoscopy-assisted colectomy versus open colectomy for treatment of non-metastatic colon cancer: a randomised trial. *Lancet* 2002; 359: 2224-9.
8. Moller CH, Steinbruchel DA. Platelet function after coronary artery bypass grafting: is there a procoagulant activity after off-pump compared with on-pump surgery? *Scand Cardiovasc J* 2003; 3: 149-53.
9. Ascione R, Williams S, Lloyd CT, *et al*. Reduced postoperative blood loss and transfusion requirement after beating-heart coronary operations: a prospective randomized study. *J Thorac Cardiovasc Surg* 2001; 121: 689-96.
10. Jayne DG, Botterill I, Ambrose NS, *et al*. Randomised clinical trial of Ligasure versus conventional diathermy for day case haemorrhoidectomy. *Br J Surg* 2002; 89: 428-32.
11. Lee WJ, Chen TC, Lai IR, *et al*. Randomised clinical trial of Ligasure versus conventional surgery for extended gastric cancer surgery. *Br J Surg* 2003; 90: 1493-6.
12. Romano F, Caprotti R, Franciosi C, *et al*. The use of Ligasure during pediatric laparoscopic splenectomy: a preliminary report. *Pediatr Surg Int* 2003; 19: 721-4.
13. Dillon A. Holmium laser prostatectomy. www.nice.org/ip138overview. November 2003.
14. Defechcreux T, Rinken F, Maweja S, *et al*. Evaluation of the ultrasonic dissector in thyroid surgery. A prospective randomised study. *Acta Chir Belg* 2003; 103: 274-7.
15. Rau HG, Wichmann MW, Schinkel S, *et al*. Surgical techniques in hepatic resections: Ultrasonic aspirator versus Jet-Cutter. A prospective randomized clinical trial. *Zentralbl Chir* 2001; 126: 586-90.
16. Takayama T, Makuuchi M, Kubota K, *et al*. Randomized comparison of ultrasonic vs clamp transection of the liver. *Arch Surg* 2001; 136: 922-8.
17. Wozniak G. Fibrin sealants in supporting surgical techniques: the importance of individual components. *Cardiovasc Surg* 2003; 11(S1): 17-21.
18. Blair SD, Jarvis P, Salmon M, McCollum C. Clinical trial of calcium alginate haemostatic swabs. *Br J Surg* 1990; 77: 568-70.
19. Jackson MR, Gillespie DL, Longenecker EG, *et al*. Hemostatic efficacy of fibrin sealant (human) on expanded poly-tetrafluoroethylene carotid patch angioplasty: a randomized clinical trial. *J Vasc Surg* 1999; 30: 461-6.
20. Brodbelt AR, Miles JB, Foy PM, Broome JC. Intraspinal oxidised cellulose (Surgicel) causing delayed paraplegia after thoracotomy - a report of three cases. *Ann R Coll Surg Engl* 2002; 84: 97-9.
21. Carless PA, Henry DA, Anthony DM. Fibrin sealant use for minimising peri-operative allogeneic blood transfusion (Cochrane Review). In: *The Cochrane Library,* Issue 1, 2004. John Wiley & Sons, Ltd., Chichester, UK.

Chapter 10

Anaesthetic Methods to Minimise Blood Loss

Philip MS Dobson BSc MB ChB FRCA

Consultant Anaesthetist, Northern General Hospital, Sheffield, UK

"The consensus of opinion is that mild hypotension (MAP 55-60mmHg) is safe and can lead to significant blood conservation in appropriate patients."

Introduction

The anaesthetist's role in blood conservation begins pre-operatively and continues through into the postoperative period. This chapter will, however, concentrate on those areas specific to the anaesthetic, i.e. deliberate hypotension, maintenance of normothermia and the effect of different fluid therapies. Other aspects are covered elsewhere in the manual.

Hypotensive anaesthesia

The use of deliberate hypotension to reduce blood loss during surgery was first advocated almost a century ago, but it did not enter clinical practice until 1946. Early techniques often employed haemorrhagic hypotension, but were associated with high complication rates! In 1948, Griffiths and Gillies [1] described hypotensive spinal anaesthesia and two years later, Enderby [2] introduced sympathetic ganglion blockade to produce hypotension.

Whilst patient positioning and meticulous anaesthetic care are important in achieving both hypotension and a "dry" surgical field, specific drug therapy may be required. It is beyond the scope of this chapter to detail their use, but techniques used include spinal and epidural anaesthesia, beta, alpha or mixed adrenergic receptor antagonists, direct acting vasodilators, sympathetic ganglion blocking agents and calcium channel blockers. The drugs can be used alone or in combination which allows lower dosages and also a reduction in side effects. For example, a beta-blocking agent can prevent the tachycardia produced by nitroprusside.

Systemic arterial pressure

Early studies that found a significant reduction in blood loss associated with hypotensive anaesthesia were poorly designed. Subsequent controlled trials, especially in orthopaedic surgery, found reductions in blood loss of around 50% [3-6]. These savings were achieved by maintaining systolic blood pressure at 80-90mmHg or mean pressure of 50-65mmHg. Blood loss was reduced in patients undergoing head, neck and intra-cranial procedures [7-8] and a retrospective study of deliberate hypotensive anaesthesia in patients undergoing radical cystectomy found a 50% reduction in blood loss [9].

Decreased bleeding correlates with the reduction in blood pressure rather than cardiac output [10], which with some agents actually increases during hypotension. Whether maintaining cardiac output during hypotension is beneficial in this context is uncertain.

Safety

The risks of hypotension have to be weighed against the perceived benefits of avoiding blood transfusion. Employing ever lower blood pressures will increase the risk of organ damage and may not achieve further reductions in blood loss. Reducing blood loss is a greater priority for patients who refuse blood transfusion and deliberate hypotension may have to be used in these patients (in addition to other blood conservation techniques) and a greater risk accepted.

In a normotensive or controlled hypertensive patient, cerebral perfusion remains adequate down to a mean arterial pressure of 50-55mmHg [11].

Patients with normal cerebral autoregulation maintain cerebral perfusion with pressures as low as 40mmHg, but levels as low as this leave no margin for error and are not recommended. Caution should also be observed when intracranial pressure is raised or cerebral autoregulation is impaired, for example in patients with a brain tumour, head injury or subarachnoid haemorrhage. In addition, during deliberate hypotension the effect of changes in $PaCO_2$ on cerebral blood flow is reduced and below a mean arterial pressure (MAP) of 50mmHg there is no response. At MAP below 60mmHg cerebral blood flow is better preserved with nitroprusside rather than with trimethaphan; hypotension produced by deep isoflurane anaesthesia also maintains cerebral oxygenation.

In patients with coronary artery disease hypotensive anaesthesia (and haemodilution [12]) must be used with caution. Appropriate monitoring to detect myocardial ischaemia is used, eg. ECG/TOE (Trans-Oesophageal Echocardiography). Vasodilating agents such as nitroprusside or nicardipine, which are used to produce hypotension tend to cause reflex tachycardia. This will adversely affect myocardial oxygen balance by both increasing demand and reducing supply. This reflex tachycardia can be controlled with an esmolol infusion, ganglion blocking agents or can be avoided by using labetalol which has both alpha-1 and beta-1 blocking properties. Agents with negative chronotropic and inotropic properties may be advantageous when used appropriately in patients with coronary artery disease. Indeed, there is level I evidence that peri-operative beta-blockade reduces cardiac morbidity and mortality.

Monitoring during deliberate hypotension

- ♦ Invasive arterial blood pressure line.
- ♦ 5-lead ECG and ST segment monitoring.
- ♦ End tidal CO_2 metering.
- ♦ Pulse-oximeter.
- ♦ Temperature probe.
- ♦ Urinary catheter (long case).
- ♦ Central venous pressure line (high blood loss anticipated).

Indications for deliberate hypotension

Blood conservation in operations normally associated with significant blood loss in "fit" patients only:

- Orthopaedics.
- Urology.
- Head, neck and intracranial surgery.

Contraindications for deliberate hypotension

- Ischaemic heart disease.
- Untreated hypertension.
- Cerebrovascular disease.
- Renal dysfunction.
- Liver dysfunction.
- Peripheral vascular disease.
- Anaemia (including deliberate).

Consideration of these contraindications should be weighed against the proposed benefits before hypotensive anaesthesia is performed. The consensus of opinion is that mild hypotension (MAP 55-60mmHg) is safe [13] and can lead to significant blood conservation in appropriate patients.

Venous pressure

Reducing venous pressure can reduce blood loss [2]. To this end patient positioning must be carefully arranged in collaboration with the surgical team.

Blood loss during laminectomy correlates with intraosseus pressure, but not systemic arterial pressure [14] and operating with the patient prone increases Inferior Vena Cava (IVC) pressure during spinal surgery when compared with the lateral position [15].

Intermittent positive pressure ventilation and positive end expiratory pressure increase blood loss compared with patients breathing spontaneously, related to a lower venous pressure in these patients. For a given systemic arterial blood pressure, the risk of cerebral ischaemia may be less in patients breathing spontaneously.

Maintenance of normothermia

Coagulation is impaired by hypothermia, which affects both platelet and clotting factor function. Even moderate hypothermia of 35.5°C increases blood loss; a core temperature above 36°C should be maintained except where hypothermia is indicated - in one study, patients undergoing total hip or knee replacement, avoiding hypothermia reduced both blood loss and blood transfusion requirements [16].

In major operations patient temperature should be closely monitored - it is possible to overheat the patient! The most accurate estimates of core temperature can be obtained from the tympanic membrane, nasopharynx, pulmonary artery or the lower oesophagus.

Aetiology of hypothermia

Vasodilatation following the induction of anaesthesia leads to a rapid shunting of heat from the core to the peripheries, lowering core temperature by approximately one degree Celsius during the first hour of anaesthesia. A further decrease in body temperature occurs as a result of radiation, convection and evaporation during surgery. This loss is proportional to the gradient between the body and ambient temperature and the extent and duration of surgery. Reflex vasoconstriction to prevent further heat loss during anaesthesia is not triggered until the core temperature is between 33°C and 35°C during general anaesthesia. Central inhibition of thermoregulation also occurs with regional anaesthesia; however, heat loss is usually less in patients having regional compared to general anaesthesia.

Methods of reducing or preventing hypothermia

Maintenance of body temperature can be achieved by reducing heat loss or by actively warming the patient. Increasing the ambient theatre temperature, exposing the patient as little as possible, limiting the duration of surgery and using minimally invasive surgical techniques all reduce heat loss. Warming all fluid and gases and applying heat via mattresses or forced air warmers are all effective.

Cutaneous warming devices

Passive insulation of the skin surface can be achieved by using cotton sheets, surgical drapes or reflective materials, i.e. "space blankets". They provide insulation by trapping a thin layer of air next to the patient. Whilst reflective drapes are marginally more efficient the different materials produce similar benefits and adding more layers has only a small additional effect. The greater the surface area uncovered the higher the heat loss. Covering the head with a cap is particularly useful in view of its high blood flow and capacity to radiate heat.

Passive insulation cannot totally prevent hypothermia during major operations - active warming devices are required. These include heated mattresses and forced air devices. Mattress heaters are themselves ineffective, largely because little heat is normally lost through the operating table, and they may actually lead to thermal burns or skin ischaemia.

Forced air blankets (eg. Warm Touch, Mallinckrodt Medical) are the most effective warming systems readily available. They are capable of maintaining normothermia during major surgery and can transfer significant quantities of heat across the skin, especially when the peripheries are vasodilated, as during most forms of anaesthesia. In contrast, in the early postoperative phase hypothermia causes reflex vasoconstriction in patients recovering from general anaesthesia and this decreases the efficiency of re-warming by impeding the transfer of heat to the core. So, it is easier to prevent intra-operative cooling than to treat postoperative hypothermia. Patients with a residual regional anaesthetic block can be re-warmed more efficiently [17].

The redistribution of body heat following induction of anaesthesia is difficult to reverse, but can be reduced if cutaneous warming is used to increase peripheral temperature prior to induction of anaesthesia or peripheral temperature is increased pre-operatively by the use of vasodilators. Keeping the legs warm is of particular importance, although they must be allowed to cool down if blood supply to the lower limbs is reduced, eg. during aortic cross-clamping. Evidence also suggests that body temperature is better preserved if invasive procedures, eg. arterial, central lines and epidurals are inserted prior to induction of anaesthesia [18].

A high ambient temperature will reduce heat loss, providing a smaller gradient for heat transfer to occur. Theatre temperatures of greater than 23°C are required to minimise heat loss in adults and even higher temperatures for small children. For staff these temperatures can be quite uncomfortable to work in and for this reason a slightly lower theatre temperature is usually maintained.

Fluid warming

Irrigation fluids and skin preparation

Many orthopaedic and urological procedures use high volumes of irrigation fluid, which if not warmed, may significantly reduce patient temperature.

Pre-operative skin preparation may reduce peripheral temperatures, which will further increase the loss of heat during the initial hour or so of anaesthesia.

Intravenous fluid

The administration of one unit of blood at 4°C or one litre of crystalloid at room temperature will decrease body temperature by up to 0.5°C. For most major operations fluid requirements will be such that if the fluid is not warmed to body temperature then a significant fall in body temperature will occur.

There are many warmers available for intravenous fluid administration; the type used is dictated by the expected fluid requirements. Fluid warming should be used for all patients receiving more than a minimal volume of fluid (eg. over 10mls/kg/hr). Simple, relatively inexpensive warming coils are sufficient for the majority of cases. For major operations where fluid administration is at a higher rate, eg. orthopaedic joint revision surgery, major bowel resection, vascular surgery or major trauma, more efficient fluid warmers are required. These systems tend to use counter-current warming and are more expensive, but generally are straightforward to use, eg. HotLine (Level 1 Inc., Rockland MA). More complex systems also include pressurising bags to enable fluid to be efficiently warmed and infused at higher rates, eg. Level One H 1000 (Level 1 Inc.). Whilst it is generally true that fluid warming alone cannot maintain normothermia, warmers such as the HotLine are very efficient and administer fluid at or slightly above 37°C.

Airway heating

In adults less than 10% of heat loss occurs through the airways. Thus, use of heat and moisture exchangers will have little impact on body temperature in adults, although the beneficial effect on airway secretions remains.

Postoperative period

Cutaneous warming methods are usually continued into the postoperative period. If high fluid requirements continue into the postoperative period, warm the fluid efficiently; this is often overlooked.

Suggested guidelines for maintaining normothermia in adults

Operation duration

<2 hours	Passive cutaneous warming
>2 hours	Active cutaneous warming

IV fluid therapy

1-3L	Simple coil warmer
>3L	HotLine
>4L/hour	Level One

High patient exposure	Active cutaneous warming eg. fracture table
High-risk patient	Lower threshold for using warming techniques

Fluid administration

Blood loss can be influenced by intravenous fluid administration. During major surgery administered fluid will lead to a progressive dilution of coagulation factors and platelets. Bleeding problems may be encountered when large volumes, eg. greater than estimated blood volume, have been infused, although the changes in coagulation will vary according to the type of fluid administered. Different crystalloids and colloids have varying effects on coagulation and potentially on blood loss. Thus, thromboelastography and clinical studies suggest that crystalloids impair haemostasis less than colloids; in fact, balanced salt solutions may cause a hypercoagulable state. Activated partial thromboplastin time decreases, and factor VIII concentration increases postoperatively in patients receiving balanced salt solution, when compared with dextran or hydroxyethyl starch.

There has been interest in the effect of different colloid solutions on coagulation. Dextrans and high molecular weight hydroxyethyl starch (HES) appear to impair coagulation significantly, which may increase blood loss. Slowly degradable medium molecular weight HES also impairs coagulation after repeated administration, whereas more rapidly degradable HES such as Voluven and gelatine-based solutions appear to have little effect [19]. A combination of gelatine or rapidly degradable HES and balanced salt solution may be optimal in avoiding blood loss due to dilutional coagulopathy [20].

Key Summary

◆ Use deliberate hypotension appropriately.
◆ Reduce venous pressure at the operative site.
◆ Maintain normothermia.
◆ Monitor coagulation if i.v. fluid requirements are greater than EBV.
◆ Be aware of the effect of different intravenous fluids on coagulation.

References

1. Griffiths HWC, Gillies J. Thoraco-lumbar splanchnicectomy and sympathectomy: anaesthetic procedure. *Anaesthesia* 1948; 3: 134-6.
2. Enderby GH. Controlled circulation with hypotensive drugs and posture to reduce bleeding during surgery. Preliminary results with pentamethonium iodide. *Lancet* 1950; 1: 1145-7.
3. Niemi TT, Pitkanen M, Syrjala M, *et al*. Comparison of hypotensive epidural anaesthesia and spinal anaesthesia on blood loss and coagulation during and after total hip arthroplasty. *Acta Anaesth Scand* 2000; 44: 457-64.
4. Barbier-Bohm G, Desmonts JM, Couderc E, *et al*. Comparative effects of induced hypotension and normovolaemic haemodilution on blood loss in total hip arthroplasty. *Br J Anaesth* 1980; 52: 1039-43.
5. Amaranath L, Cascorbi HF, Singh-Amaranath AV, *et al*. Relation of anaesthesia to total hip replacement and control of operative blood loss. *Anesth Analg* 1975; 54: 641-8.
6. Qvist TF, Skovsted P, Sorenson MB. Moderate hypotensive anaesthesia for reduction of blood loss during total hip replacement. *Acta Anaesth Scand* 1982; 26: 351-3.
7. Blau WS, Kafer ER, Anderson JA. Esmolol is more effective than sodium nitroprusside in reducing blood loss during orthognathic surgery. *Anesth Analg* 1992; 75: 172-8.
8. Diaz JH, Lockhart CH. Hypotensive anaesthesia for craniectomy in infancy. *Br J Anaesth* 1979; 51: 233-5.
9. Ahlering TE, Henderson JB, Skinner DG. Controlled hypotensive anaesthesia to reduce blood loss in radical cystectomy for bladder cancer. *J Urol* 1983; 129: 953-4.
10. Sivarajan M, Amory DW, Everett GB. Blood pressure not cardiac output determines blood loss during induced hypotension. *Anesth Analg* 1980; 59: 203-6.
11. Sharrock NE, Salvati EA. Hypotensive epidural anaesthesia for total hip arthroplasty. *Acta Orthop Scand* 1996; 67: 91-107.

12. Crystal GJ, Salem MR. Myocardial and systemic haemodynamics during isovolaemic haemodilution alone and combined with nitroprusside induced controlled hypotension. *Anesth Analg* 1991; 72: 227-37.

13. Williams-Russo P, Sharrock NE, Mattis S, *et al.* Randomised trial of hypotensive epidural anaesthesia in older adults. *Anesthesiol* 1999; 91: 926-35.

14. Kakiuchi M. Intraoperative blood loss during cervical laminoplasty correlates with the vertebral intraosseous pressure. *J Bone Joint Surg* 2002; 84: 518-20.

15. Lee TC, Yang LC, Chen HJ. Effect of patient position and hypotensive anaesthesia on inferior vena caval pressure. *Spine* 1998; 23: 941-7.

16. Schmied H, Kurz A, Sessler DI, *et al.* Mild intraoperative hypothermia increases blood loss and allogeneic transfusion requirements during total hip arthroplasty. *Lancet* 1996; 347: 289-92.

17. Szmuk P, Ezri T, Sessler DI, *et al.* Spinal anaesthesia speeds active postoperative rewarming. *Anesthesiol* 1997; 87: 1050-4.

18 Stoneham M, Howell S, Neill F. Heat loss during induction of anaesthesia for elective aortic surgery. *Anaesthesia* 2000; 51: 79-82.

19. de Jonge E, Levi M. Effects of different plasma substitutes on blood coagulation: a comparative review. *Crit Care Med* 2001; 29: 1261-67.

20. Spahn D, Casutt M. Eliminating blood transfusions: new aspects and perspectives. *Anesthesiol* 2000; 93: 242-55.

Chapter 11

Pharmacological Approaches

Roger Cordery FRCA
Fellow, Anaesthesia
David Royston FRCA
Consultant Anaesthetist
Harefield Hospital, Harefield, UK

"The current gold standard for prevention of transfusion after cardiac surgery is high-dose aprotinin."

Pharmacological adjuncts to good surgical haemostasis can prove invaluable in high-risk patients, causing a reduction not only in the use of blood (packed red cells), but also in the use of haemostatic blood components.

The main groups of patients where these drugs may be of most benefit are those where there is an expected high level of transfusion requirements (i.e. those undergoing cardiac, hepatic transplantation and major trauma and orthopaedic surgery). This is reflected in the various studies to date, and the different groups will be considered in turn.

Available agents

The drugs used most commonly in reduction of autologous transfusion are the serine protease inhibitors, such as aprotinin (Trasylol®), the lysine analogue anti-fibrinolytics, ε-aminocaproic acid (Amicar®) and tranexamic acid (Cyclokapron®) and DDAVP (Desmopressin®). More recently, activated recombinant factor VIIa (rFVIIa) (NovoSeven®) has become available.

Aprotinin

Aprotinin is a naturally occurring, basic polypeptide, obtained commercially from bovine lungs which forms reversible complexes with nearly all the serine protease molecules involved in coagulation and fibrinolysis; this inhibition is dose-dependent [1]. Its role in nature is unknown.

Cardiac surgery

Prevention of red cell transfusion

The current gold standard for prevention of transfusion after cardiac surgery is high-dose aprotinin. The original dose regimen was to give a bolus of 2×10^6 KIU of aprotinin over about 20 minutes prior to surgery and a similar amount into the oxygenator prime together with an infusion of 500,000 KIU every hour. This regimen can be simplified as a weight-related dose of 40,000 KIU (4mL).kg^{-1} as the loading dose with the same amount into the oxygenator and no infusion [2]. A meta-analysis reported by Laupacis and colleagues (the International Study of Perioperative Transfusion [ISPOT] group) [3] of patients undergoing cardiac surgery, showed a consistent, significant benefit of using aprotinin in not only primary operations, but also in predictably higher risk procedures such as re-operation and patients taking aspirin.

Similarly, the conclusions of a systemic review by the Cochrane group [4] showed that aprotinin therapy reduced the rate of transfusion by 30%. However, the data for this review included a variety of regimes, some of which were probably sub-therapeutic. It also included a wide variety of cardiac surgical procedures (revascularisation, valve replacement, surgery with circulatory arrest and cardiac transplantation), where a higher than expected average rate of transfusion was noted in some of the patients allocated to placebo groups. This suggests that procedures with a higher innate risk of transfusion may have been included in the aprotinin studies, thereby potentially skewing the data.

Prevention of need for haemostatic components

Haemostatic component therapy represents up to 80% of transfusion requirements in patients undergoing resternotomy. Using aprotinin in these higher-risk patients causes a dose-dependent reduction in postoperative blood loss [1], to the extent where the need for haemostatic component transfusion may be eliminated [5]. This effect is unique amongst currently available interventions, and has been used as part of an integrated approach to avoid transfusion in re-operative cardiac surgery in those patients of the Jehovah's Witness faith [6].

Other potential benefits

A meta-analysis by Levi and colleagues [7] of patients undergoing cardiac surgery showed a two-fold decrease in mortality from 2.8% to 1.6% (a relative risk reduction of 0.55 [95% CI 0.34-0.90]) in those receiving high-dose aprotinin. Rates of resternotomy for bleeding were also reduced from about 3% to nearly zero.

Hepatic surgery

Initial reports of the use of aprotinin in hepatic transplantation were conflicting. However, the European Multicentre Study of the use of Aprotinin in Liver Transplantation (EMSALT) allowed a randomised, placebo-controlled evaluation [8]. They used high-dose aprotinin, regular dose aprotinin and placebo. Total transfusion requirements were 37% lower in the higher-dose group (loading dose of 2×10^6 KIU at induction of anaesthesia, followed by a continuous infusion of 1×10^6 KIU.hr^{-1} and an additional 1×10^6 KIU at 30 minutes before reperfusion), and 20% lower in the regular dose (loading dose of 2×10^6 KIU at induction of anaesthesia followed by a continuous infusion of 500.000 KIU.hr^{-1} and no extra bolus) group than with placebo. The apparent dose-response relationship is similar to that seen in cardiac surgery.

Orthopaedic/trauma surgery

Two randomised placebo-controlled studies of high-dose aprotinin during primary hip replacement showed a reduction in the need for allogeneic transfusion [9], but there appeared to be no dose-response relationship. The effect was not uniformly seen, possibly reflecting the use of other methods of red cell conservation known to be of benefit in orthopaedic surgery.

In higher-risk operations such as hip replacements where the joint is infected or invaded by tumour, there was a significant dose-dependant reduction in transfusion [10]. The 18 patients given the higher dose of a load of 4 x10^6 KIU over 20 minutes followed by 1 x10^6 KIU .hr^{-1} received a total of seven units of donor red cells. This compares with the 101 units of donor red cells given to the 18 patients in the placebo group.

Aortic surgery

Despite initial enthusiasm [11], prospective randomised placebo controlled trials have shown aprotinin to be of no benefit in elective aortoiliac reconstruction [12] or emergency surgery for ruptured aortic aneurysm [13].

Lysine analogue anti-fibrinolytics

These drugs act by attachment to the lysine-binding site on plasminogen, thereby inhibiting its activation of fibrinolysis.

Cardiac surgery

Reduction of red cell transfusion

Despite a number of studies reporting that use of these drugs reduces drain losses after primary cardiac surgery, they do not seem to consistently reduce the need for allogeneic blood transfusion.

Two meta-analyses did show some overall benefit of tranexamic acid use [3], and one amalgamated study of both analogues [4] showed a reduction in red cell transfusion. However, these conclusions are subject to several caveats:-

♦ The studies included non-cardiac (orthopaedic and liver transplantation) surgery.
♦ The data for reduction in blood transfusion were obtained from only three studies of patients undergoing cardiac surgery.
♦ For tranexamic acid use, there was no reduction in transfusion requirements in patients taking aspirin pre-operatively and no consistent benefit used in re-operation.

♦ The transfusion benefit seen with tranexamic acid was most powerful when used in open-label studies, and in blinded prospective placebo-controlled trials, the effect was neither universal nor consistent.
♦ There was no dose-response effect seen with tranexamic acid. This is consistent with previous studies [14] where a plateau effect was observed for drain loss reduction at a dose of $10mg.kg^{-1}$ load and an infusion of $1mg.kg^{-1}.hr^{-1}$. There was, however, no consistent effect to reduce transfusion requirements at any dose administered.

Both the meta-analyses [3,4] failed to demonstrate any statistically significant effect of ε-aminocaproic acid, at any dose, on the amount of allogeneic blood transfusion required.

Preventing the need for haemostatic components

The only placebo-controlled study in the literature comparing the effects of the lysine analogues did not show any statistically significant effect of these agents on the need for haemostatic blood components [15].

Other efficacy end points

Unlike the data for aprotinin, the relative risk for mortality was not reduced in 11 placebo-controlled studies of lysine analogues [7]. Despite reported reductions in drain losses, the rate of resternotomy was not significantly reduced, being about 3% for placebo and treated groups. There are at present no reports suggesting a role for the use of the lysine analogues in patients of the Jehovah's Witness faith.

Hepatic surgery

Trials of anti-fibrinolytics have not shown any consistent reduction in transfusion requirements during liver transplantation. Fibrinolysis during the anhepatic phase of transplantation is inhibited by tranexamic acid, but without effect on packed cell transfusion [16]. Very high-dose tranexamic acid (20g) has been shown to reduce intra-operative transfusion of both red cells and components [17]. The authors of this article expressed some concern about potential thrombotic complications at this dose level and co-administered heparin and dipyridamole with this regimen. Similarly, a comparison of a high-dose tranexamic acid (5g) regimen with ε-aminocaproic acid (8g) and placebo, concluded that tranexamic acid, but not ε-aminocaproic acid, reduced intra-operative but not total transfusions of red cells or haemostatic products [18].

Orthopaedic/trauma surgery

The most consistent support for the use of tranexamic acid in orthopaedic surgery comes from data for its application in knee surgery associated with tourniquet use. A recent prospective randomised study shows a significant reduction in red cell transfusion using oral and intravenous tranexamic acid in total knee replacement [19]. In addition, there is some limited but inconsistent data suggesting a reduction in red cell transfusion during hip surgery. In children undergoing scoliosis repair, use of tranexamic acid in conjunction with acute normovolaemic haemodilution and a haemoglobin concentration trigger of 7g/dl, does show a significant reduction in total transfusion (donor and cell salvage), but not in donor transfusions alone [20]. As with other studies, the use of tranexamic acid has not been shown to have an effect on haemostatic component use.

DDAVP (Desmopressin)

Cardiac surgery

Initial interest in the use of DDAVP stemmed from a trial in 1986 suggesting a positive benefit from its use in high-risk surgical procedures. However, further investigation and use failed to support this in the cardiac patient [5].

There has been a resurgence of interest in DDAVP following studies that suggest some benefit in patients with acquired platelet dysfunction, such as those with uraemia or those taking aspirin. There has also been one case report of its use in a patient taking ticlopidine.

Hepatic and orthopaedic/trauma surgery

Currently, there are no data to show any benefit of the use of DDAVP during liver transplantation or resection. There has also been no benefit shown in orthopaedic surgery. However, there is little specific data relating to its use in patients taking aspirin or non-steroidal anti-inflammatory drugs pre-operatively, and this may warrant further investigation.

rFVIIa (NovoSeven®)

This is the recombinant form of human factor VIIa. It was initially developed to treat bleeding in patients with haemophilia known to have inhibitors to factors VIII or IX (around 15-25% of this population) [21]. The currently recommended dose to achieve this is about $90\mu g.kg^{-1}$. Early studies showed that it reduced bleeding into muscle (in 82%) and joints (in 89%) of patients. In a randomised controlled trial [22] in surgical patients with inhibitors, a bolus of $35\mu g.kg^{-1}$ or $90\mu g.kg^{-1}$ was repeated every two hours for 48 hours and then at 2-6 hourly for three further days. Satisfactory haemostasis was achieved in all 14 patients allocated to the higher dose and 12 of the 15 in the lower dose.

The results of rFVIIa use in the above population have led to an explosion of interest in its use elsewhere. There have been several anecdotal reports of its use in patients without haemophilia who received this as rescue therapy for life-threatening haemorrhage in major trauma. The outcome of these reports suggests that rFVIIa may have a specific role in such circumstances. This compound has also been used successfully in patients with congenital platelet dysfunction. At the time of writing however, randomised trial data that support the use of NovoSeven have yet to be published.

Safety issues

The major concern with the use of these agents is thrombosis. Levi et al [7] showed no significant increase in the incidence of myocardial infarction in 18 trials, nor did the Cochrane review [4]. Similarly, for the lysine analogues, no statistically significant difference was seen in the incidence of myocardial infarction in six trials.

The incidence of stroke after cardiac surgery has been shown to be reduced with high-dose aprotinin therapy, a finding supported by the

Cochrane review [4]. However, there may be a trend towards an increased risk of stroke with tranexamic acid use based on the data included in the Cochrane study, although this may reflect a low incidence of stroke in the control group patients.

Thrombotic risk has not been formally evaluated with rFVIIa in humans. It has been shown to reduce both the Activated Partial Thromboplastin Time (APTT) and the Prothrombin Time (PT), which although of potential benefit in anticoagulated patients, may represent a prothrombotic state. This may be particularly true in Disseminated Intravascular Coagulation (DIC), atherosclerotic disease, crush injury patients or patients with septicaemia who are already predisposed to a higher risk of thrombosis.

The second major problem is one of hypersensitivity. With aprotinin use, this seems to be reduced to nearly zero if aprotinin re-exposure occurs after an interval of more than six months. The incidence may be as high as 20% for a shorter time interval [23].

NovoSeven is contraindicated in patients allergic to murine, hamster and bovine proteins, which may be present as contaminants of the manufacturing process.

Key Summary

◆ High-dose aprotinin reduces red cell and component transfusion in cardiac, hepatic transplant and major orthopaedic, but not vascular surgery.

◆ Tranexamic acid has inconsistent effects to reduce red cell and no effect on component transfusion.

◆ Tranexamic acid has no proven benefit for patients taking antiplatelet therapy.

◆ Epsilon aminocaproic acid does not reduce allogeneic transfusion.

◆ DDAVP after cardiac surgery may be useful in proven platelet dysfunction.

◆ There are no reports for efficacy of rFVIIa from randomised placebo controlled studies outside the primary licensed indication. Anecdotal reports suggest a benefit in trauma.

◆ None of the agents appear to be effective in orthopaedics, which may reflect the success of other blood conservation strategies.

◆ There are no adequately powered placebo controlled studies to evaluate the safety of either the lysine analogues or rFVIIa.

References

1. Royston D. Aprotinin versus lysine analogues: the debate continues. *Ann Thorac Surg* 1998; 65(4 Suppl): S9-19.
2. Royston D, Cardigan R, Gippner-Steppert C, Jochum M. Is perioperative plasma aprotinin concentration more predictable and constant after a weight-related dose regimen? *Anesth Analg* 2001; 92(4): 830-6.
3. Laupacis A, Fergusson D. Drugs to minimize perioperative blood loss in cardiac surgery: meta-analyses using perioperative blood transfusion as the outcome. The International Study of Peri-operative Transfusion (ISPOT) Investigators. *Anesth Analg* 1997; 85(6): 1258-67.
4. Henry DA, Moxey AJ, Carless PA, *et al*. Anti-fibrinolytic use for minimising perioperative allogeneic blood transfusion. *Cochrane Database Syst Rev* 2001(1): CD001886.
5. Kovesi T, Royston D. Pharmacological approaches to reducing allogeneic blood exposure. *Vox Sang* 2003; 84(1): 2-10.
6. Rosengart TK, Helm RE, DeBois WJ, Garcia N, Krieger KH, Isom OW. Open heart operations without transfusion using a multimodality blood conservation strategy in 50

Jehovah's Witness patients: implications for a "bloodless" surgical technique. *J Am Coll Surg* 1997; 184(6): 618-29.

7. Levi M, Cromheecke ME, de Jonge E, *et al.* Pharmacological strategies to decrease excessive blood loss in cardiac surgery: a meta-analysis of clinically relevant endpoints [see comments]. *Lancet* 1999; 354(9194): 1940-7.

8. Porte RJ, Molenaar IQ, Begliomini B, *et al.* Aprotinin and transfusion requirements in orthotopic liver transplantation: a multicentre randomised double-blind study. EMSALT Study Group [see comments]. *Lancet* 2000; 355(9212): 1303-9.

9. Murkin JM, Haig GM, Beer KJ, *et al.* Aprotinin decreases exposure to allogeneic blood during primary unilateral total hip replacement. *J Bone Joint Surg Am* 2000; 82(5): 675-84.

10. Samama CM, Langeron O, Rosencher N, *et al.* Aprotinin versus placebo in major orthopedic surgery: a randomized, double-blinded, dose-ranging study. *Anesth Analg* 2002; 95(2): 287-93.

11. Thompson JF, Roath OS, Francis JL, Webster JH, Chant AD. Aprotinin in peripheral vascular surgery. *Lancet* 1990; 335(8694): 911.

12. Ranaboldo CJ, Thompson JF, Davies JN, Shutt AM, Francis JN, Roath OS, Webster JH, Chant AD. Prospective randomized placebo-controlled trial of aprotinin for elective aortic reconstruction. *Br J Surg* 1997; 84(8): 1110-3.

13. Robinson J, Nawaz S, Beard JD. Randomized, multicentre, double-blind, placebo-controlled trial of the use of aprotinin in the repair of ruptured abdominal aortic aneurysm. On behalf of the Joint Vascular Research Group. *Br J Surg* 2000; 87(6): 754-7.

14. Horrow JC, Van Riper DF, Strong MD, Grunewald KE, Parmet JL. The dose-response relationship of tranexamic acid. *Anesthesiology* 1995; 82(2): 383-92 .

15. Hardy JF, Belisle S, Dupont C, *et al.* Prophylactic tranexamic acid and epsilon-aminocaproic acid for primary myocardial revascularization. *Ann Thorac Surg* 1998; 65(2): 371-6.

16. Kaspar M, Ramsay MA, Nguyen AT, Cogswell M, Hurst G, Ramsay KJ. Continuous small-dose tranexamic acid reduces fibrinolysis but not transfusion requirements during orthotopic liver transplantation. *Anesth Analg* 1997; 85(2): 281-5.

17. Boylan JF, Klinck JR, Sandler AN, *et al.* Tranexamic acid reduces blood loss, transfusion requirements, and coagulation factor use in primary orthotopic liver transplantation. *Anesthesiology* 1996; 85(5): 1043-8.

18. Dalmau A, Sabate A, Acosta F, *et al.* Tranexamic acid reduces red cell transfusion better than epsilon-aminocaproic acid or placebo in liver transplantation. *Anesth Analg* 2000; 91(1): 29-34.

19. Ellis M, Zohar E, Ifrach N, Stern A, Sapir O, Fredman B. Oral tranexamic acid in total knee replacement; results of a randomised study. *Vox Sang* 2004; 87 (3): 50.

20. Neilipovitz DT, Murto K, Hall L, Barrowman NJ, Splinter WM. A randomized trial of tranexamic acid to reduce blood transfusion for scoliosis surgery. *Anesth Analg* 2001; 93(1): 82-7.

21. Hedner U. Recombinant factor VIIa (Novoseven) as a hemostatic agent. *Semin Hematol* 2001; 38(4 Suppl 12): 43-7.

22. Shapiro AD. Recombinant factor VIIa in the treatment of bleeding in hemophilic children with inhibitors. *Semin Thromb Hemost* 2000; 26(4): 413-9.

23. Dietrich W, Spath P, Zuhlsdorf M, *et al.* Anaphylactic reactions to aprotinin reexposure in cardiac surgery: relation to antiaprotinin immunoglobulin G and E antibodies. *Anesthesiology* 2001; 95(1): 64-71.

Chapter 12

Postoperative cell salvage

Andrew Hamer MB ChB MD FRCS(Orth)

Consultant Orthopaedic Surgeon, Northern General Hospital, Sheffield, UK

"... re-infusing blood salvaged from wound drains stimulates the production of natural killer cell precursors and hence may upregulate the immune system ..."

Introduction

Postoperative cell salvage is established in certain areas of surgical practice almost as routine. There are significant advantages in the reduction of postoperative allogeneic blood transfusion and the associated reduction in transfusion associated complications.

The technique relies on the collection of blood shed in the postoperative period into wound drains, which is then either filtered and returned to the patient, or washed before retransfusion.

The technique has developed to this stage largely by the availability of simple, cost-effective equipment. Early devices were often too complex for routine use, or risked the introduction of infection by inefficient connections within the drainage circuits.

Indications

Postoperative cell salvage techniques are effective where there is a predictable postoperative blood loss, and where that blood is relatively "clean". The volume of blood required for the technique to be justified is approximately 400ml or more, but this loss should occur within six hours of wound closure. This length of time is chosen as the safe period during which blood can be safely returned to the patient with the minimum risk of complications.

Postoperative cell salvage has traditionally been used in cardiac and orthopaedic surgery, especially total knee arthroplasty. There are approximately 45,000 total knee replacements performed in the UK each year, with a mean blood loss of 800ml. Use of tourniquets can reduce intra-operative loss, most occurring in the postoperative period [1].

The quality of blood lost after total knee replacement is high, as it often results from brisk bleeding from cancellous bone after the operation, which settles with time. This clean postoperative blood loss is not contaminated, and is ideal for retransfusion.

There is considerable worldwide variation in postoperative transfusion practice after total knee replacement, but assuming the initial haemoglobin is satisfactory, and that any blood lost is retransfused, the need for allogeneic blood can be considerably reduced or indeed eliminated. Within orthopaedic surgery, postoperative cell salvage could initially be used for the following specific indications:

- Elective total knee replacement (unilateral or bilateral).
- Spinal surgery with large exposures.
- Hip and knee revision arthroplasty surgery (but not for infection).

Conditions for use, and contraindications are listed in Tables 1 and 2.

Problems

The passage of blood through wound drainage tubing, filters and valves risks haemolysis and the production of free haemoglobin. Excessive free haemoglobin and in particular, red cell stroma, can be toxic to the glomeruli, and lead to renal impairment. In practical terms, this does not seem to be a problem in clinical practice if the volumes of retransfused

Table 1. Conditions for use of postoperative cell salvage.

- ◆ Suitable indication, no contraindication.
- ◆ Technique discussed with the patient in advance and documented.
- ◆ Strict sterility, following the manufacturer's instructions.
- ◆ Salvaged blood must not be retransfused more than six hours after the start of collection (or in accordance with local transfusion policy).
- ◆ A 40-micron blood filter must be used during re-infusion.
- ◆ The patient will require intravenous fluid in addition to the salvaged blood.

Table 2. Contraindications for use of postoperative cell salvage.

- ◆ Contamination of the surgical field by betadine, chlorhexidine, hydrogen peroxide, antibiotics or other agents not for parenteral use. (NB. The use of these agents intra-operatively is not a contraindication to postoperative cell salvage providing adequate lavage of the wound using saline is performed prior to closure.)
- ◆ Surgical team, anaesthetists or nursing staff unfamiliar with the use of the technique.
- ◆ The patient declines the use of the technique.
- ◆ Patients with sickle cell disease, trait and other red cell disorders.
- ◆ The presence of infection or malignancy in the operative field (possibly).

blood are less than 1000ml (although this is an arbitrary figure). Systems that wash shed blood may allow larger volumes to be retransfused, as in this process the majority of the free haemoglobin is removed.

Wound drainage fluid may be diluted with wound irrigation fluid, and may therefore have relatively low haemoglobin in comparison with circulating blood [2]. The introduction of a leucocyte-reducing filter into the retransfusion circuit reduces the drained blood haemoglobin even further.

In cardiac surgery, the presence of cardiac enzymes in non-washed drain blood may confuse the clinical picture after retransfusion.

It is vital that all staff that use retransfusion equipment are familiar and confident with its use. It is important that "occasional" use is avoided, as mistakes could be made unnecessarily increasing the risks to the patient.

Techniques

Postoperative cell salvage devices are divided into those that leave the blood products unwashed, and those that wash the drained blood.

Unwashed systems

These systems are simple adaptations of existing wound drainage equipment. Standard wound drainage tubes are attached to a reservoir that is held at a negative pressure, often with a coarse pre-filter in place to remove large fat globules, bone debris, etc. The vacuum is either maintained by attachment to existing hospital suction, by plastic bellows, or by self-contained vacuum pumps. Once the reservoirs have filled to approximately 300-400ml, the blood is decanted into blood bags directly from the drainage container, without interrupting the closed system.

Blood is then re-infused to the patient through a standard 40 micron blood filter. European Commission and American Association of Blood Banks guidelines recommend collection and re-infusion procedures to be finished within six hours after wound closure in view of the theoretical risk of bacterial contamination, and subsequent risk of septicaemia, although this timeframe may be less in some centres.

Examples of a battery operated device and bellows devices are shown in Figures 1 and 2.

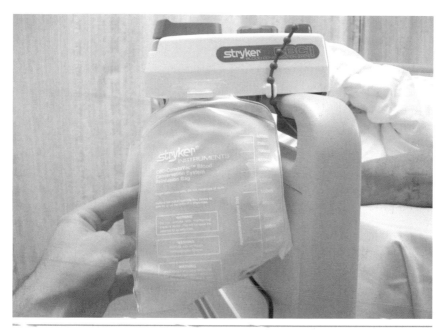

Figure 1. Constavac™ re-infusion device (courtesy of Stryker Corporation).

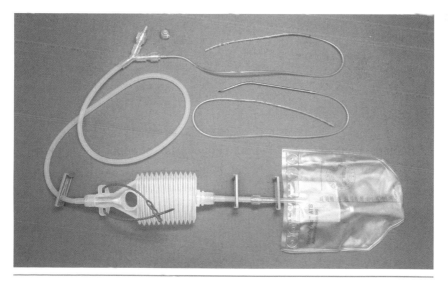

Figure 2. Bellows operated retransfusion device (courtesy of Unomedical Ltd).

Washed systems

The technology used in intra-operative cell salvage systems has been developed for use in postoperative cell salvage. These newer systems are capable of being used as intra-operative cell savers, and can then be attached to the drainage tubes to collect blood postoperatively. Blood collected in this manner is centrifuged to remove plasma and excess fluid, and the concentrated red blood cells are washed with saline before being retransfused to the patient. The haematocrit of the re-infused blood is higher (approx 75%) than with unwashed systems (20-30%). The advantage of this technique is that larger volumes of blood can be returned to the patient than with unwashed systems, but the time during which retransfusion can be carried out is usually the same, at six hours from wound closure. The device is more bulky than those that do not wash the drained blood, and has to be transported on a drip stand. However, its operation is simple, with most operations being automated. An example of such a device is shown in Figure 3.

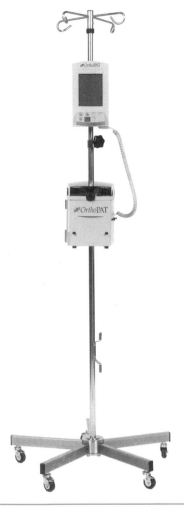

Figure 3. Orthopat™ washed blood intra-operative/postoperative cell salvage device (courtesy of Haemonetics Ltd.).

Evidence

Effect on postoperative transfusion practice

Postoperative cell salvage reduces the need for allogeneic blood transfusion. Groh *et al*, in a relatively small study found that the use of the Solcotrans device reduced the number of patients requiring allogeneic blood following total knee replacement from ten out of 25 (40%) to two out of 25 (8%). The haematocrit of the scavenged blood was 29.3% using this unwashed system [3]. No evidence of coagulopathy, thrombocytopenia, or renal dysfunction was found.

Jensen *et al* demonstrated that shed blood is defibrinated and that re-infusion of unwashed blood did not change the coagulative capacity of the patients [4].

The blood requirements in a group of patients undergoing bilateral simultaneous total knee replacement were reduced from a mean of 6.3 to 3.8 units with no adverse events, and no transfusion reactions in the retransfused group [5].

Experience with postoperative cell salvage at the author's institution in a group of 56 patients was associated with no need for allogeneic blood transfusion in 44 (78%) of patients. The mean volume of blood retransfused in this group was 493ml per patient, equivalent to approximately 1.5 units of banked blood.

Cost-effectiveness

Determining whether postoperative cell salvage is cost-effective depends upon local circumstances:

- How much is charged for allogeneic blood per unit?
- How much allogeneic blood is saved using cell salvage?
- What is the cost difference between the cell salvage devices and existing wound drains?

At the author's institution, blood is charged at approximately $\in$ 200 per unit. On the basis of 1.5 units of blood being saved per patient ($\in$ 300) and the cost of the device ($\in$ 184), the technique is cost-effective.

Immune and inflammatory consequences of unwashed blood

Retransfusion of shed blood collected after operation has become popular, but reports of side effects led to a search for possible causes. Unwashed wound drainage blood collected after operation contains levels of pro-inflammatory mediators that can account for these reported side effects. Higher levels of histamine and PGE_2 in shed blood have been found in drained blood compared with venous blood [6]. Dalen *et al* investigated whether leucocyte-reducing filters influenced complement activation and the formation of pro-inflammatory cytokines in autotransfusion drain blood after knee arthroplasty. A leucocyte filter was placed in the drainage circuit and reduced IL-8 and TNF-α in drain blood, but at the same time triggered complement activation [2].

On the other hand, recent work has demonstrated that re-infusing blood salvaged from wound drains stimulates the production of natural killer cell precursors and hence, may upregulate the immune system. Salvaged blood reversed immunosuppression caused by surgery and blood loss. This could partly explain the clinical benefit observed in recipients of autologous blood [7].

Practicalities

The introduction of postoperative cell salvage into routine practice can be difficult. As the appropriate cases for the technique are, by definition, common, it is likely that a large number of staff will be affected with such a change in practice. The best way to introduce such a new technique is to have the support of representatives of all the areas in the hospital where the devices will be used. These include:

- Surgeons.
- Anaesthetists.
- Haematologists.

- Operating theatre staff.
- Recovery room staff.
- Ward staff.

All will have to be persuaded that postoperative cell salvage has many advantages. Local audits can be powerful in demonstrating the benefits to patients. Hospital managers will be persuaded by the powerful benefit/cost ratio!

Any manufacturer supplying postoperative autotransfusion devices should provide comprehensive education for all staff, as part of the procurement process. This should include a representative of the company being present at the introduction of the devices, giving presentations to the appropriate staff groups, and visiting the site regularly once the devices become established.

Key Summary

- Postoperative cell salvage is safe, economic and clinically beneficial.
- Selective introduction can reduce requirement for banked blood.
- Modern devices are simple to use.
- Techniques available are cost-effective.
- Introduction into routine practice requires a multi-disciplinary approach.
- Training input is important from equipment manufacturers.

References

1. Abdel-Salam A, Eyres KS. Effects of tourniquet during total knee arthroplasty. A prospective randomised study. *J Bone Joint Surg* 1995; 77-B (2): 250-3.

2. Dalen T, Bengtsson A, Brorsson B, Engstrom KG. Inflammatory mediators in autotransfusion drain blood after knee arthroplasty, with and without leucocyte reduction. *Vox Sang* 2003; 85: 31-39.

3. Groh GI, Buchert PK, Allen WC. A comparison of transfusion requirements after total knee arthroplasty using the Solcotrans autotransfusion system. *Journal of Arthroplasty* 1990; 5(3): 281-5.

4. Jensen CM, Pilegaard R, Hviid K, Nielsen JD, Nielsen HJ. Quality of reinfused drainage blood after total knee arthroplasty. *Journal of Arthroplasty* 1999; 14(3): 312-8.

5. Breakwell LM, Getty CJM, Dobson P. The efficacy of autologous blood transfusion in bilateral total knee arthroplasty. *The Knee* 2000; 7 (3): 145-149.

6. Mottl-Link S, Russlies M, Klinger M, Seyfarth M, Ascherl R, Gradinger R. Erythrocytes and proinflammatory mediators in wound drainage. *Vox Sang* 1998; 75(3): 205-11.

7. Gharehbaghian A, Haque KMG, Truman C, Evans R, Morse R, Newman J, Bannister G, Rogers C, Bradley BA. Effect of autologous blood on postoperative natural killer cell precursor frequency. *Lancet* 2004; 363: 1025-30.

Chapter 13

Transfusion Triggers in Surgical and Critically Ill Patients

Timothy S Walsh BSc(Hons) MB ChB(Hons) MRCP FRCA MD
Consultant in Anaesthetics and Critical Care
New Edinburgh Royal Infirmary, Edinburgh, Scotland, UK

"Start with the assumption that restrictive transfusion triggers are safe. A trigger of 70-80g/L is supported by clinical evidence."

Introduction

The lowest acceptable haemoglobin concentration in surgical and critically ill patients is the level at which the risk associated with anaemia outweighs the risks of blood transfusion. This concentration is often used as a transfusion trigger. Ideally, at these concentrations blood transfusion should result in measurable improvements in the patient that justify the decision to transfuse. It is self-evident that the transfusion trigger used may strongly influence the exposure of individual patients to allogeneic red blood cells. Unfortunately, the lowest acceptable haemoglobin is not a simple physiological parameter.

This chapter will review briefly the physiological role of blood in oxygen transport, the normal response to anaemia and the balance between oxygen supply and demand. From this basis the evidence regarding what haemoglobin value is acceptable will be reviewed, concluding with an evidence-based appraisal of what transfusion triggers should be used in surgical and critically ill patients.

The role of red cells in oxygen delivery

Oxygen delivery (DO_2) is the amount of oxygen delivered to the body from the heart. It is the product of cardiac output (CO) and the oxygen content of arterial blood (CaO_2) and is usually expressed in mL.min^{-1}:

$$DO_2 = CO \times CaO_2$$

The oxygen content of arterial blood (CaO_2) is described using the equation:

$$CaO_2 = (k_1 \times Hb \times SaO_2) + (k_2 \times PaO_2)$$

where Hb is the haemoglobin concentration (g/L), SaO_2 is the arterial Hb oxygen saturation and PaO_2 is arterial oxygen partial pressure. In health >98% of oxygen is bound to Hb. The oxygen combining capacity of Hb is represented by the constant k_1 above. In theory, each gram of Hb binds 1.39mL of O_2. However, in practice, the presence of abnormal forms of Hb, such as carboxyhaemoglobin and methaemoglobin, reduce the oxygen combining capacity of Hb to 1.31mL/g. The constant k_2 represents the solubility coefficient of oxygen in plasma. Normal arterial oxygen content is about 200mL/L, and normal adult oxygen delivery about 1000mL/minute. It follows that anaemia significantly decreases DO_2 unless there is a compensatory increase in cardiac output.

The normal physiological response to anaemia

When patients become anaemic a physiological response occurs to maintain oxygen delivery to the tissues. If an adequate circulating intravascular volume is maintained, these compensatory mechanisms are as follows:

♦ *Increased cardiac output.* Anaemia reduces blood viscosity, which decreases the resistance to blood flow peripherally. This increases venous return and facilitates left ventricular emptying by decreasing afterload. The net effect is an increase in cardiac output. Sympathetic activation also occurs which may increase heart rate and/or myocardial contractility, but these play a minor role in increasing the cardiac output of a normal heart in anaemia as long as normovolaemia is maintained.

♦ *Increased oxygen extraction by the tissues.* Normal body oxygen consumption is about 250mL/minute and the oxygen extraction ratio is 0.25. Redistribution of blood flow to areas of high demand, such as the myocardium and the brain, improve overall oxygen extraction rates. In the microcirculation, red blood cells normally lose oxygen as they travel through the arterial tree, but in the anaemic state blood flow is increased and the pre-capillary oxygen loss is reduced making more oxygen available for areas of high demand. Normovolaemic anaemia has little effect on the capillary haematocrit because this is normally very low due to "plasma skimming". The "normal" capillary haematocrit has been estimated at approximately 8.5%.

The oxygen supply and demand balance

In health

The oxygen transport system normally operates to maintain constant oxygen consumption, even if DO_2 varies widely. If global DO_2 decreases, oxygen extraction increases in an attempt to maintain an adequate oxygen supply. If DO_2 continues to decrease a point is reached where the oxygen extraction ration cannot increase further. This point is called the "critical DO_2", and it is the point below which energy production in cells becomes limited by the supply of oxygen. The critical DO_2 could result from low cardiac output or low arterial oxygen content or a combination of these factors. If the decrease in DO_2 is due to anaemia in the presence of normal circulating volume, the Hb concentration at the critical DO_2 is termed the "critical Hb concentration". Any further reduction in DO_2 will result in tissue hypoxia, conversion to anaerobic metabolism and may cause tissue damage. The critical DO_2 is not a fixed value, but varies between organs and is dependent on the metabolic activity of the tissue. The value for critical DO_2 has been estimated at about $4mL.kg^{-1}minute^{-1}$ in humans [1]. The value for the critical haemoglobin concentration in health is of considerable interest; it represents an absolute lower limit of anaemia, which should be avoided even in otherwise healthy individuals. The critical haemoglobin value for healthy individuals has been estimated at about 50g/L based on the following evidence:

♦ A series of experiments in healthy volunteers and in surgical patients were carried out using normovolaemic haemodilution [2]. At an Hb concentration of 50g/L, heart rate, stroke volume, and cardiac output were increased, but oxygen delivery was decreased. Despite this, calculated oxygen consumption (VO_2) and plasma lactate concentration remained relatively unchanged. Overall, this degree of severe anaemia was well tolerated, but there were subtle effects on cognitive function and a small number of individuals developed asymptomatic ST-segment depression on the electrocardiograph.

♦ Various published case reports, mainly describing patients refusing transfusions on religious grounds, found that haemoglobin concentrations of 40-50g/L can be tolerated [3].

During critical illness

Tissue hypoxia is common during critical illness. Early studies suggested that many critically ill patients had an inadequate DO_2 because when DO_2 was increased by blood transfusions, fluids or inotropic drugs, the VO_2 also increased. This implied that VO_2 was dependent on DO_2 over a much wider range than normal and that there was a persistent tissue oxygen debt. This was termed "pathological oxygen supply dependency". However, many of these studies were complicated by methodological problems and many were detecting physiological, rather than pathological, supply dependency [4].

Recent work shows that pathological oxygen supply dependency is less common and less severe than previously thought in most clinically resuscitated critically ill patients. Abnormal oxygen extraction capabilities do exist in critically ill patients, particularly in organs such as the gut that has a circulation prone to hypoxia. This means that the critical haemoglobin may be different during critical illness than in health, particularly for some organs. At present, there are no reliable monitors that indicate inadequate DO_2 or haemoglobin concentration in sick patients, and no widely applicable specific physiological parameters that indicate when blood transfusion is indicated [3].

Transfusion triggers

The appropriate transfusion trigger for an individual patient needs to take into account several factors:

♦ Why is this patient anaemic and what is the erythropoietic response likely to be?

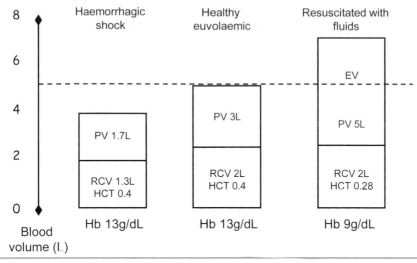

Figure 1. The relationship between red cell volume, plasma volume, and haemoglobin concentration during haemorrhage, healthy euvolemia, and fluid resuscitation with clear fluids. PV = plasma volume; RCV = red cell volume; HCT = haematocrit; Hb = haemoglobin concentration; EV = excess volume.

♦ What do clinical studies and trials indicate are acceptable safe levels of haemoglobin in these patients?
♦ What factors should modify the transfusion triggers used in individual patients?

Why do critically ill patients become anaemic?

Haemodilution

Patients frequently receive large volumes of crystalloid or colloid solutions during peri-operative management or during resuscitation. This is appropriate and evidence-based because using fluids to optimise cardiac preload is central to strategies that also optimise peri-operative DO_2 and are associated with improved outcome [5]. In addition, the increasing use of epidural anaesthesia for major surgery is associated with vasodilatation. Haemoglobin concentration or haematocrit are measures made relative to plasma volume; they are not reliable estimates of red cell mass (Figure 1).

A low postoperative haemoglobin may occur despite normal red cell mass and rapidly return to normal during the days following surgery, particularly when epidural anaesthesia is discontinued. This corresponds to loss by diuresis of the "excess volume" of clear fluid given during surgery.

Blood loss

It is important to estimate the relative contribution of blood loss to a low haemoglobin concentration, particularly in the context of the effect of haemodilution described above. Sources of blood loss include the following:

♦ Operative blood loss.
♦ Postoperative blood loss from operation sites.
♦ Blood sampling. It has been estimated that patients in intensive care lose 40mL per day in diagnostic blood sampling. Daily volumes are highest during the first 24 hours.
♦ Occult blood loss. During critical illness significant blood loss can occur from extracorporeal circuits, intravascular catheter sites, or from the gastrointestinal tract.

Reduced red cell production

The normal response to anaemia is release of erythropoietin from the kidney and increased bone marrow erythropoiesis. Recent evidence indicates that the inflammatory response to surgery and critical illness results in an abnormal erythropoietic response [6]. This is characterized by:

♦ An inappropriately low circulating erythropoietin concentration for the degree of anaemia;
♦ Iron indices that are similar to those found in the "anaemia of chronic disease", namely low serum iron, total iron binding capacity, transferrin, transferrin saturation, and serum iron/total iron binding capacity ratio, but a normal or increased serum ferritin. These findings collectively indicate functional iron deficiency.
♦ A lack of reticulocyte response.

The reason for these abnormalities is incompletely understood, but is probably a consequence of inflammatory processes. The state has been termed the "acute" anaemia of chronic disease. It is probably present in most critically ill patients, but also occurs in response to the inflammatory response to major surgery. Factors influencing the duration of marrow suppression are not well understood, but may include the magnitude of the inflammatory response and the presence of complications, such as infection. Pre-existing anaemia associated with chronic disease is also relevant.

Clinical trials of transfusion thresholds

Effect of blood transfusions on indices of tissue hypoxia and oxygenation

Studies in critically ill patients have investigated whether blood transfusions improve indices of tissue oxygenation such as global oxygen consumption, plasma lactate and acid-base status. High quality studies found no evidence of improvement in these indices when the baseline haemoglobin concentration was 80-100g/L [3]. Although currently available oxygenation indices lack sufficient sensitivity and specificity, these studies support transfusion triggers of 70-80g/L for most patients.

Randomised trials of transfusion triggers in surgical and critically ill patients

A Cochrane systematic review is the best available synthesis of evidence [7]. It found:

♦ Insufficient studies of the subject.
♦ Restrictive transfusion triggers do not adversely affect mortality for most surgical and critically ill patients. A transfusion trigger of 70-80g/L is at least as safe as higher values, and may be preferable.
♦ Restrictive transfusion triggers decrease the number of patients exposed to blood transfusions and the numbers of blood transfusions used.
♦ Insufficient evidence for patients with ischaemic heart disease, and recommended caution in these groups.

♦ Insufficient evidence concerning outcomes other than mortality, such as fatigue and functional status.

♦ The conclusions are strongly influenced by a single large study in critically ill patients, the Transfusion Requirements in Critical Care (TRICC) study.

The TRICC study

This study compared two transfusion thresholds for patients admitted to Canadian intensive care units whose haemoglobin concentration was 90g/L or less within 72 hours of ICU admission [8]. Patients were randomised to receive single unit red cell transfusions either at a transfusion trigger of 100g/L (to maintain haemoglobin concentration 100 to 120g/L) (liberal group) or at a trigger of 70g/L (to maintain haemoglobin at 70 to 90g/L) (restrictive group). The intervention lasted throughout ICU stay. The main outcome measure was 30-day mortality.

The study was stopped after 838 patients were enrolled because of slow recruitment. The original study design was for 1620 patients to detect a 5% difference in 30-day mortality. Key findings were:

♦ Mean haemoglobin concentrations in the restrictive group were 85g/L (mean 2.5 red cell units per admission) compared with 107g/L in the liberal group (mean 5.2 red cell units per admission).

♦ Red cell use in the restrictive transfusion group was 54% lower than in the liberal group.

♦ There was a trend towards lower 30-day mortality in the restrictive group (23.3% versus 18.7%, p=0.11).

♦ For patients with lower illness severity (APACHE II score <20) restrictive practice was associated with significantly lower 30-day mortality (8.7% versus 16.1%, p=0.02).

♦ For younger patients (aged <55 years) restrictive practice was associated with significantly lower 30-day mortality.

♦ Cardiac complications were more common in the liberal strategy group, including the incidence of new myocardial infarction (12 versus three cases; p<0.02).

♦ Shortcomings of the study included selection bias - many patients were excluded by their physicians.

The TRICC study is the strongest evidence that sick patients tolerate anaemia well and that maintaining a haemoglobin concentration of 70-90g/L can significantly decrease blood use without adversely affecting mortality. The data support the hypothesis that some patients may have adverse outcomes associated with liberal blood transfusions. A possible confounder in the study interpretation was that blood was not leucodepleted.

What factors should be considered when deciding the transfusion trigger for an individual patient?

Acute factors

Acute factors that may decrease an individual patient's tolerance to anaemia are listed in Table 1. In an individual patient this list can be used to assess the balance of oxygen supply and demand and aid decisions regarding the appropriate transfusion threshold.

Chronic factors

Ischaemic heart disease

Patients with ischaemic heart disease may be less tolerant of anaemia and require higher transfusion triggers [9]. There is inadequate high quality evidence for this patient group, but the following support a higher transfusion trigger than for patients without evidence of ischaemic heart disease [9]:

- Animal studies indicate that coronary stenosis decreases tolerance of the heart to anaemia.
- The heart has a high coronary oxygen extraction ratio and has less capacity than other organs to compensate for reduced arterial oxygen content.
- Cohort studies indicate that critically ill and surgical patients with ischaemic heart disease have adverse outcomes compared with similar patients without ischaemic heart disease at haemoglobin levels below 90-100g/L [10,11].

Table 1 Factors that influence oxygen supply and demand in surgical and critically ill patients.

Factors that may compromise oxygen delivery

♦ Hypovolaemia
♦ Impaired cardiac function

- Acute ischaemia
- Acute myocardial infarction
- Acute valvular disorders
- Acute cardiomyopathies, eg. sepsis

♦ Reduced oxygen carrying capacity

- Anaemia

Factors associated with high tissue oxygen demand

♦ Major surgery, trauma, burn injury
♦ Severe acute inflammatory illnesses, eg. pancreatitis
♦ Sepsis
♦ Pyrexia
♦ Shivering
♦ Seizures
♦ Agitation/anxiety/pain

♦ A Cochrane systematic review of evidence concerning transfusion triggers found insufficient evidence to make strong recommendations for patients with ischaemic heart disease and advised caution in using very restrictive transfusion triggers [7].

In practice, the best method to assess the appropriate transfusion trigger for a patient with ischaemic heart disease should include:

♦ Assessment of the severity of the coronary disease.
♦ Monitoring for signs of acute cardiac dysfunction or ischaemia, (modern monitoring offers multiple lead electrocardiography with automated S-T segment analysis).

♦ Assessment of the systemic oxygen demand (high demand will increase cardiac work).
♦ Assessment of coronary perfusion/flow. Coronary perfusion is most likely to be decreased by tachycardia (reducing diastolic flow time) and low diastolic blood pressure (reducing the perfusion pressure).

Current recommendations are:

♦ Anaemic surgical and critically ill patients with stable mild/moderate ischaemic heart disease should be managed with a transfusion trigger of 70-80g/L maintaining haemoglobin in the 70-90g/L range until anaemia recovers.
♦ For patients with severe disease a transfusion trigger of 90g/L should be considered.
♦ For patients with acute coronary syndromes or acute myocardial infarction, a transfusion trigger of 100g/L should be considered.

The evidence supporting liberal use of transfusions in patients with severe disease is not from large randomised studies

Chronic lung disease

Patients with chronic lung disease may have hypoxaemia and/or hypercapnia. In these patients tolerance of anaemia may be decreased. There is little evidence to indicate whether a higher transfusion trigger is appropriate for these patients compared with patients without lung disease. Some small observational studies suggest that critically ill patients with chronic lung disease are more likely to wean from ventilation after transfusion [3]. Sub-group analysis of the TRICC trial found a trend towards shorter ventilation times with restrictive transfusion triggers for patients requiring over seven days mechanical ventilation in the intensive care unit [12].

Cerebrovascular disease

There is insufficient evidence to make evidence-based recommendations for these patients, but intuitively, the same approach as that towards patients with coronary disease would seem sensible.

Volume of blood transfusion in response to transfusion triggers

The most frequent red blood cell prescription in response to a low haemoglobin concentration without evidence of bleeding is two units of red cell concentrate/packed red cells. There is no evidence to support this practice. Depending on individual processing practices and the size of the patient, each unit increases haemoglobin concentration by 5-10g/L. Good clinical practice should be to decide the desired increment in haemoglobin, estimate the likely increment per unit in the individual patient, and prescribe individual units to specifically achieve the change. Near patient methods for measuring haemoglobin concentration are widely available in many hospitals; checking haemoglobin concentration after each red cell unit may decrease unnecessary transfusions.

Suggested best practice for managing postoperative haemoglobin concentration

An algorithm for assessing and managing haemoglobin concentration in surgical and critically ill patients is shown in Figure 2. Key steps in this process are:

♦ Start with the assumption that restrictive transfusion triggers are safe. A trigger of 70-80g/L is supported by clinical evidence.
♦ Assess volume status. If hypovolaemia is present, efforts should concentrate on restoring circulating volume rather than the value of haemoglobin concentration.
♦ Once intravascular volume status is adequate and peripheral perfusion is restored (judged by clinical signs or monitoring), the individual transfusion trigger should be determined by consideration of:

• Oxygen supply-demand balance at that time using indices of tissue hypoxia (acid-base status, lactate).
• Myocardial status.

♦ Clearly document the agreed transfusion trigger for a patient in the clinical record. This will guide other staff who may need to make transfusion decisions with less knowledge of the patient.

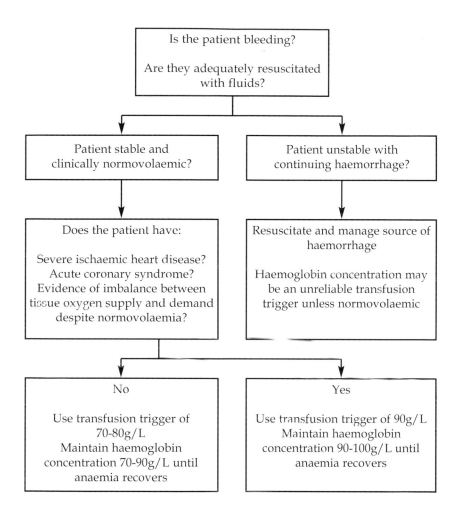

Figure 2. A simple algorithm for assessing and managing red cell transfusion triggers in surgical and critically ill patients.

♦ Document the reason for transfusion if this occurs (a medicolegal requirement).
♦ Use single unit red cell transfusions, unless there is haemorrhage.
♦ Reassess each patient regularly. Look for evidence that should change the transfusion trigger such as:

- Myocardial ischaemia.
- Signs of tissue hypoxia.

Evidence-based guidelines

A number of evidence-based guidelines for transfusion in critically ill and peri-operative patients have been produced:

♦ Peri-operative blood transfusion for elective surgery: A National Clinical Guideline. www.sign.ac.uk 2003.
♦ Handbook of Transfusion Medicine. www.transfusionguidelines.org.uk 2003.

Key Summary

◆ Haemoglobin concentration should be used to determine transfusion requirement in conjunction with assessment of circulating red cell volume, cardiac output, and the oxygen demand by tissues.

◆ In normovolaemic patients a transfusion trigger of 70-80g/L is safe.

◆ Transfusions should be used to maintain haemoglobin concentrations of 70-90g/L for most patients until anaemia recovers.

◆ If the patient is not bleeding, single unit transfusions should be prescribed followed by reassessment of haemoglobin concentration.

◆ Patients with ischaemic heart disease may not tolerate severe anaemia; the evidence base for this group is weak, but transfusion thresholds of 90g/L are recommended.

◆ Patients with acute coronary syndromes should have a transfusion threshold of 90-100g/L.

◆ Document the agreed transfusion trigger clearly in the patient record and reassess it regularly if the patient's condition changes.

References

1. Ronco JJ, Fenwick JC, Tweeddale MG, Wiggs BR, Phang PT, Cooper DJ, et al. Identification of the critical oxygen delivery for anaerobic metabolism in critically ill septic and nonseptic humans. JAMA 1993; 270(14): 1724-30.

2. Weiskopf RB, Viele MK, Feiner J, Kelley S, Lieberman J, Noorani M, et al. Human cardiovascular and metabolic response to acute, severe isovolemic anemia. JAMA 1998; 279(3): 217-21.

3. McLellan SA, McClelland DB, Walsh TS. Anaemia and red blood cell transfusion in the critically ill patient. Blood Rev 2003; 17(4): 195-208.

4. Walsh TS. Recent advances in gas exchange measurement in intensive care patients. Br J Anaesth 2003; 91(1): 120-31.

5. Heyland DK, Cook DJ, King D, Kernerman P, Brun-Buisson C. Maximizing oxygen delivery in critically ill patients: a methodologic appraisal of the evidence. *Crit Care Med* 1996; 24(3): 517-24.

6. Corwin HLM. Anemia of the critically ill: "acute" anemia of chronic disease*. *Crit Care Med* 2001; 29(9): Supplement-S200.

7. Hill SR, Carless PA, Henry DA, Carson JL, Hebert PC, McClleland DBL, Henderson KM. Transfusion thresholds and other strategies for guiding allogeneic red blood cell transfusion (Cochrane Review). In: *The Cochrane Library,* Issue 2, 2002. Update Software, Oxford.

8. Hebert PC, Wells G, Blajchman MA, Marshall J, Martin C, Pagliarello G, *et al.* A multicenter, randomized, controlled clinical trial of transfusion requirements in critical care. Transfusion Requirements in Critical Care Investigators, Canadian Critical Care Trials Group. *N Engl J Med* 1999; 340(6): 409-17.

9. Walsh TS, McClelland DB. When should we transfuse critically ill and perioperative patients with known coronary artery disease? *Br J Anaesth* 2003; 90(6): 719-22.

10. Hebert PC, Wells G, Tweeddale M, Martin C, Marshall J, Pham B, *et al.* Does transfusion practice affect mortality in critically ill patients? Transfusion Requirements in Critical Care (TRICC) Investigators and the Canadian Critical Care Trials Group. *Am J Respir Crit Care Med* 1997; 155(5): 1618-23.

11. Carson JL, Duff A, Poses RM, Berlin JA, Spence RK, Trout R, *et al.* Effect of anaemia and cardiovascular disease on surgical mortality and morbidity. *Lancet* 1996; 348(9034): 1055-60.

12. Hebert PC, Blajchman MA, Cook DJ, Yetisir E, Wells G, Marshall J, *et al.* Do blood transfusions improve outcomes related to mechanical ventilation? *Chest* 2001; 119(6): 1850-7.

Chapter 14

Management of Transfusion on the Ward

Magnus Garrioch MB ChB (Birm) FRCA FRCP (Glasg.)

Consultant in Anaesthesia and Intensive Care

Part-time Senior Lecturer

Southern General Hospital & University of Glasgow, Glasgow, UK

"Optimal use of blood products on the wards is desirable both for patient safety and the efficient use of a precious and exhaustible resource."

Introduction

The management of blood products on the ward is of paramount importance due to concerns regarding both the safety and the costs of transfusing blood. Sixty percent of red cell transfusions occur on the ward [1]. Mismatched blood transfusion continues to be reported annually as the commonest cause of transfusion-related morbidity and mortality [1]. For this reason it is important to have robust mechanisms in place for ensuring that ward transfusion practice is done well.

There are a number of approaches available to achieve best practice regarding postoperative and other ward-based blood transfusions:

♦ Timely and accurate measurement of haemoglobin.
♦ Rational blood usage policies.
♦ Education and audit of practice.
♦ Bloodless medicine.

Although it makes sense to ensure that blood is only used when necessary, anaemia carries serious and possibly life-threatening consequences. A balance must be struck to ensure that blood is used wisely.

Accurate measurement of haemoglobin

This is the goal of the clinical team when faced with either a bleeding or an anaemic patient. Blood transfusion requirements rely on haemoglobin measurement. A number of methods are available.

Laboratory testing

Haemoglobin measurement necessitates drawing a blood sample into a correctly labelled container and sending the sample to the haematology laboratory. Haemoglobin concentration is routinely measured by using automated counters, which work by converting haemoglobin, methaemoglobin and carboxyhaemoglobin into cyanmethaemoglobin (HiCN) using potassium cyanide and potassium ferricyanide. HiCN has a specific light absorbance and this is then measured at 540nm [2]. Hyperlipaemia and high white cell counts may occasionally interfere with the analysis but the technique has become the "gold standard".

Most modern machines also employ a secondary light scatter technique as a means of verifying the light absorbance. The sample flows through a very small aperture, of such a diameter that only one red cell can pass at a given time. A focused beam of light is passed through the tube. When a red cell passes through the light beam, light is scattered off the cell and is detected by a number of photo-optical detectors. The degree of scatter is related to both the size of the cell and the number of cells in the sample, so those cells can be both counted and sized. Counters of this variety (Coulter® counters) are calibrated daily and are subject to tight quality control.

Although laboratory-based testing is accepted as ideal, it may not be fast enough in the case of a rapidly bleeding patient. Examples are patients suffering from major haemorrhage due to major trauma or an obstetric catastrophe. Under these circumstances two potential problems may result from a clinical team estimating blood loss.

♦ Inappropriate transfusion may be given to replace perceived blood loss.

♦ In the converse situation of an underestimation of blood loss, blood can be withheld inappropriately.

The first scenario leads to over-transfusion, whereas the second can lead to a potentially dangerous anaemia. Near patient testing can avoid these problems.

Near patient testing

Accurate and rapid estimations of haemoglobin level, clotting and a range of other assays, can be performed at the bedside by "near patient testing". These methods can be useful when clinicians are practising at remote sites without access to a haematology laboratory. Rapidly changing clinical situations, such as in the operating room or trauma bay, make near patient testing an attractive option.

The HemoCue®

The HemoCue is a small device (height 90mm, width 160mm, depth 210mm, weight 250g) which can be battery or mains operated. It is easily transported and is simple to use. The method for determination of plasma haemoglobin is based upon an optical measuring cuvette of small volume and short light path. The sample is drawn into the cuvette by capillary action where it mixes with the appropriate reagents. The cuvettes for the HemoCue contain sodium desoxychrolate to haemolyse red cells, sodium nitrite to convert haemoglobin to methaemoglobin and sodium azide to convert methaemoglobin to haemoglobinazide which is then measured spectrophotometrically. The absorbance of the sample is read at 570nm and 880nm to compensate for turbidity in the sample. The transmittance is read every five seconds until a steady state is obtained. The haemoglobin concentration is calculated according to a programmed algorithm and displayed within 45 seconds. The calibration of the instrument is checked daily with a reference cuvette.

The accuracy of the device depends upon the operator. Air bubbles in the sample or excess blood on the back of the cuvette can lead to erroneous results. When sampling from bottles rather than a fingerprick, insufficient mixing of the sample may also lead to errors. Squeezing of the site of fingerprick leads to inaccuracy as does leaving the sample too long before analysis.

The HemoCue has shown to be accurate when compared with Coulter machines [3], but it is important that staff are correctly trained and a quality control programme is mandatory. The HemoCue should not replace laboratory testing for all samples but is a useful adjunct when managing patients with rapidly changing circumstances.

Centrifugal haematocrit analysis

The StatCrit device is an example of a small centrifuge that can spin manual haematocrit samples and so obtain an estimate of the haemoglobin concentration. A fingerprick sample of blood is drawn into a fine capillary tube whose end is sealed with putty. The tube is centrifuged at 12,000 rpm for three minutes. The capillary tube is read against a scale where the haematocrit and derived haemoglobin concentration are read off.

The technique has some risks. Blood spillage or fracture of the glass tubes may occur. This may endanger staff and potentially contaminate equipment.

Conductivity and adjusted conductivity

Haemoglobin molecules have electrical charge by virtue of the presence of iron so the conductivity of a sample is proportional to the haemoglobin concentration. The method is accurate under average conditions [4], but not when serum electrolytes and/or protein concentrations deviate from normal, such as during haemodilution [5]. An adjusted conductivity haemoglobin estimate can be obtained by correcting for changes in non-red cell constituents. This technique is not particularly useful in clinical practice.

Rational blood usage policies

It is good practice to develop policies for blood usage in any hospital. This can be done for a number of different scenarios.

Sudden blood loss on the ward

Development of a major haemorrhage protocol to co-ordinate clinical staff, portering staff and laboratory staff is invaluable. The hospital switchboard can act as a co-ordinating centre to optimise management of an unexpected major haemorrhage.

In most hospitals, Group O negative blood is available in the transfusion department and at strategic places such as the obstetric unit, accident and emergency department and emergency theatre suites. Type-specific blood is very safe and can be life-saving - the Rhesus group is irrelevant for male patients and for females who are either beyond childbearing age or who do not wish to have children.

Advanced Trauma Life Support (ATLS©) guidelines developed by the American College of Surgeons suggest transfusion of blood after an initial 2L volume of crystalloid if an estimated blood loss of greater than 40% of the blood volume (2L in a 70kg adult) has occurred [6]. This restores circulating volume and prevents critical tissue hypoxia occurring due to sudden anaemia. ATLS© also suggest that blood will almost certainly be necessary when a blood loss of 30% (1.5L) has occurred or in cases of ongoing haemorrhage. Sudden catastrophic blood loss should lead to patient transfer to an operating room as soon as possible. A suitably trained surgeon should be available to control the haemorrhage. Resuscitation should not delay this transfer but should occur concurrently with it.

If there is likely to be delay in surgical intervention to stop the haemorrhage, resuscitation should be limited to a systolic blood pressure of 90mm mercury (Hg) [7]. This prevents over-resuscitation leading to dilution of clotting factors and also clot displacement from a bleeding point. Both these factors promote further haemorrhage.

In acute haemorrhage:

◆ Blood ordering should be considered early in the resuscitation process.
◆ Surgical control is mandatory and should be performed as soon as possible.
◆ Fluid resuscitation should be carefully managed, particularly before surgical control has been achieved.
◆ Investigations should not delay surgical exploration.
◆ The safest place for the patient is in the operating room!

Guidelines for transfusion

General hospital practice

It is difficult to change established medical practice. Simply issuing a statement or letter to clinicians based on recent research or evidence is not effective at implementing change [8]. Five steps are suggested to influence behaviour:

◆ Audit of local practice. Clinicians are often surprised by how much blood has been ordered compared to how much has actually been used.
◆ Peer group presentation of best evidence including recent research and discussion of the audited current practice. Comparison with either another institution or another healthcare system is appropriate to stimulate discussion.
◆ Introduction of a guideline with suitable publicity and "policing" of that guideline.
◆ Total red cell pack utilisation and crossmatched to transfused ratios should be sent to a lead clinician who can influence practice (include business managers in the circulation list).
◆ Re-audit after a pre-determined period to establish whether a change in practice has occurred and present it to the target audience again.

This cycle should be regularly reviewed by the Hospital Transfusion Committee; although the process is time-consuming it can have very encouraging results.

Development of national guidelines can assist greatly in promoting sensible blood use and steps should be taken to promote them. National guidelines have been in existence for some time but are not always implemented. Reasons why this happens are a failure to communicate the guideline, a lack of faith in the guideline or a failure to understand how the guideline can be applied to the particular patient groups under the clinician's care. Clinical governance meetings should help to inform clinicians but often a local guideline, together with a motivated group of professionals, can help to encourage a change in practice. Wide discussion and promotion of the guideline before introduction gives a chance for concerns to be voiced and allows supplemental evidence to be supplied to sceptics. Audit of practice before the introduction of the guideline adds extra opportunity for discussion and helps promote the relevance of the suggested practice to individual clinical teams. Such a guideline was designed for use in a 1000-bed Scottish hospital and is shown in Figure 1.

Implementing a guideline and auditing its compliance provides a powerful educational tool. In the quoted case, the initial audit recorded a number of variables: the number of red cell packs issued; number returned; when a red cell transfusion occurrod; patient details; and the location of the transfusion. When blood was given, the haemoglobin level of patients transfused before and after the transfusion episode was cross-referenced. Comments written on the request form were recorded. Blood requested and subsequently returned unused was also documented.

The results were fed back to all clinical groups within the hospital and the audit cycle was repeated 12 months later. This process showed where blood was being used, suggested reasons why blood was being given and for what transfusion threshold. Each division of the hospital was prompted to think closely about how blood use could be improved.

Red cell transfusions were reduced by 20% over the one-year period [9]. No demonstrable morbidity or mortality was demonstrated by this practice change.

This guideline promotes best practice regarding blood use within the Southern General Hospital. Recent audit revealed widespread differences in practice and confusion as to when and how to prescribe blood.

Indications for transfusion

1. Acute blood loss

An acute blood loss of greater than 20% of blood volume (about 1000mls blood) will often need a transfusion. Do not delay ordering blood in situations where blood loss is acute and rapid. If blood loss is very rapid, the hospital's Major Haemorrhage Protocol should be activated by dialling 3333.

2. For surgical patients

Consider transfusion if:
- Pre-operative haemoglobin is less than 80g/L and the surgery is associated with the probability of major blood loss.
- Postoperative haemoglobin falls below 70g/L.
- Pre-operative anaemia MUST be investigated, as medical management may be more appropriate than transfusion.

3. Anaemia in active myocardial infarction (Hb below 100g/L)

These patients are among the few who may benefit from a Hb above 80. Transfusion to an Hb of 100g/L is acceptable but to overshoot to 110 may be excessive. Evaluate effect of each unit as it is given.

4. Anaemia in other patients (Hb below 100g/L but above 70g/L)

Consider transfusion in normovolaemic patients ONLY if they have symptomatic anaemia. Symptoms and signs of anaemia include:
- Shortness of breath for no other reason.
- ST depression on ECG.
- Angina.
- Tachycardia for no other reason.
- Syncope/postural hypotension.

Transfusion above 100g/L is very rarely indicated and WILL be questioned by haematology staff.

- Think before transfusion. Blood is expensive and potentially dangerous if used inappropriately.
- Reassess after each unit is given. Do you need to give more?
- Stop if symptoms/signs shown above resolve.
- Stop if you have reached an adequate Hb, i.e. above 80g/L in symptomless patients (100g/L in acute MI).

Figure 1. Guidelines for blood transfusion and accompanying flow chart. *Reproduced with the permission of South Glasgow University Hospitals NHS Trust.*

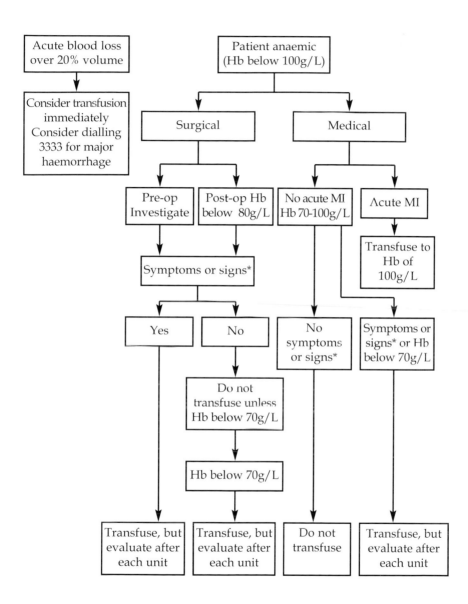

Figure 1. *continued.* Haemoglobin = Hb; pre-operative = pre-op; postoperative = post-op; myocardial infarction = MI; electrocardiogram = ECG; * symptoms/signs, see point 4.

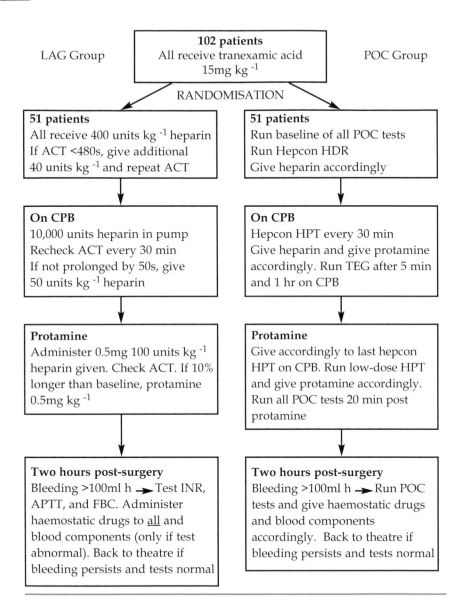

Figure 2. Management of laboratory algorithm guided (LAG) and point of care (POC) groups. ACT = activated clotting time; CPB = cardiopulmonary bypass; INR = international normalised ratio; APTT = activated thromboplastin time; FBC = full blood count; HDR = heparin dose response; TEG = thromboelastography; HPT = heparin protamine titration. *Reproduced with permission* [11].

Cardiac surgical practice

The use of guidelines or algorithms in cardiac surgery also can lead to a beneficial effect on practice. Cardiac surgery is a heavy user of blood products. In the north of England, 4.1% of all packed red cell transfusions are used for coronary artery bypass surgery [10].

An example of what can be achieved by adherence to an algorithm has been demonstrated in one centre (Figure 2) [11]. By employing a trigger haemoglobin and routine use of coagulation tests, postoperative cardiac surgical transfusion rates were compared to a group where "clinical judgement" was used. Transfusion rates were reduced from 85% to under 70% by adoption of the algorithm, although there was no significant difference in the postoperative blood loss between groups. Initiatives should be continued to ensure standards are maintained [12].

Bloodless medicine on the wards

The European Commission recently pointed out that optimal blood usage should be viewed as an essential component of blood safety [13]. Many interventions can minimise the use of blood on the wards. Many techniques are relevant to the immediate postoperative period. These include close surveillance for bleeding, adequate oxygenation, restricted phlebotomy for diagnostic tests, postoperative cell salvage, pharmacological enhancement of haemostasis, avoidance of hypertension, tolerance of normovolaemic anaemia, and meticulous management of anticoagulants and antiplatelet agents.

When encouraging a reduction in the use of blood, a balanced approach is necessary. Blood transfusion is still a very safe procedure. Limiting postoperative transfusion has not been subject to large-scale clinical trials to quantify relative risk. These trials are needed to answer questions such as the relationship between postoperative rehabilitation after hip replacement and mild anaemia, compared with a higher haemoglobin level. Although there are small risks with blood transfusion, the risk of a major morbid event due to acute anaemia, eg. myocardial infarction, must be remembered.

Close observation of blood loss

Unexpected or unexplained blood loss should always be investigated and promptly treated. Early return to theatre must be considered; there is a great risk in adopting the "it will probably stop" attitude. Local protocols should be held by ward nurses to ensure that haemorrhage is recognised and treated. Surgical haemostasis should always be the ultimate aim. Where further surgery is not indicated, then coagulopathy should be promptly treated with the help of the laboratory.

Oxygen therapy

Supplemental oxygen can be given to counter the effects of low haemoglobin. This remains one of the principles of immediate resuscitation. In an acute blood loss situation, 100% oxygen (or as near to it as possible) should be given via a trauma mask.

Restriction of phlebotomy

This is considered elsewhere but deserves amplification. Tests should be restricted to those that are absolutely necessary. Most hospitals have come to an agreement with anaesthetic departments and, indeed, the Royal College of Anaesthetists has produced guidelines to restrict blood testing. Microtest cuvettes are available from companies such as Beckton-Dickinson and are invaluable for patients who require long-term blood sampling, such as those on the intensive care unit, or in paediatric practice.

Iron therapy

Oral iron is effective, but the tablets are unpalatable and have a wide variety of side effects. Tarry stools, dyspepsia and constipation are common associated complaints, particularly in the elderly and thus compliance with iron therapy is often poor. Intravenous iron is recommended under circumstances where postoperative haemoglobin levels are low and blood transfusion is refused. Increased erythropoietic effects (4.5-5 times that of basal erythrocyte production) are achievable but the effect only lasts for 7-10 days. After the erythropoietic effect is saturated, further iron is deposited in the reticuloendothelial system and is potentially hazardous. Intravenous iron therapy should only be carried out with the assistance of a transfusion medicine specialist.

Erythropoietin (EPO)

EPO is a glycoprotein produced principally by the kidney and is a major stimulant for production of red cells. Recombinant EPO is used to boost postoperative haemoglobin levels to good effect [14]. Side effects such as hypertension and thrombotic events are uncommon in surgical patients receiving the drug for a short time, but the main limitation of EPO use is its cost. It is recommended that supplemental iron is administered to maximise red cell production. It is unlikely that EPO will ever be used routinely but it is useful in some circumstances. Female patients with rheumatoid disease who may have low blood volume, or Jehovah's Witness patients who have refused blood, are two common groups that receive EPO.

Conclusions

Many different methods may be employed to optimally manage postoperative haemoglobin levels in a ward setting. Accurate and timely recording of haemoglobin concentration, then acting on it in an educated way optimises the use of blood transfusion on the ward. Auditing adherence to guidelines is an effective tool in achieving the important balance between using blood when it is needed and preventing unnecessary transfusion when it is not. Future use of intravenous iron and erythropoietin may become more common due to either the increasing cost, or decreased availability, of red cells or if patients increasingly refuse blood products.

Key Summary

◆   Many interventions can minimise the use of blood on the wards:

- Close surveillance for bleeding.
- Adequate oxygenation.
- Restricted phlebotomy for diagnostic tests.
- Postoperative cell salvage.
- Pharmacological enhancement of haemostasis.
- Avoidance of hypertension.
- Tolerance of normovolaemic anaemia.
- Management of anticoagulants and antiplatelet agents.

◆   Laboratory-based testing is the "gold standard" for haemoglobin measurement.

◆   Accurate estimates of haemoglobin levels, clotting and other assays can be performed at the bedside (near patient testing) with appropriate staff training.

◆   ATLS guidelines suggest transfusion of blood after an initial 2L volume of crystalloid if an estimated blood loss of greater than 40% of the blood volume (2L in a 70kg adult) has occurred.

◆   National local guidelines can assist in promoting sensible blood use.

References

1. The Serious Hazards of Transfusion Committee. SHOT Annual Report 2000-2001. SHOT, Manchester, 2002.
2. *Practical haematology.* Churchill Livingstone, Edinburgh, 1991.
3. Lardi AM, Hirst C, Mortimer AJ, McCollum CN. Evaluation of the HemoCue® for measuring intra-operative haemoglobin concentrations: a comparison with the Coulter Max-M®. *Anaesthesia* 1998; 53: 349-52.

4. Kernen JA, Wurzel H, Okada R. New electronic method for measuring haematocrit: clincal evaluation. *Journal of Laboratory Clinical Medicine* 1961; 57: 635-41.

5. McNulty SE, Sharkey SJ, Asam B, Lee JH. Evaluation of STAT-CRIT haematocrit determination in comparison to Coulter and centrifuge: the effects of isotonic hemodilution and albumin administration. *Anesthesia & Analgesia* 1993; 76: 830-4.

6. American College of Surgeons. Advanced Trauma Life Support for Doctors (ATLS). Instructor Course Manual. Chicago, 1997.

7. Bickell WH, Wall Jr MJ, Pepe PE, Martin RR, Ginger VF, Allen MK, *et al*. Immediate versus delayed fluid resuscitation for hypotensive patients with penetrating torso injuries. *New Engl J Med* 1994; 331(17): 1105-9.

8. Lomas J. Words without action? The production, disemination and impact of consensus recommendations. *Annual Review of Public Health* 1991; 12: 41-65.

9. Garrioch MA, Sandbach J, Pirie E, Morrison A, Todd A, Green R. Reducing red cell transfusion by audit, education and a new guideline in a large teaching hospital. *Transfus Med* 2004; 1491: 25-31.

10. Wells AW, Mounter PJ, Chapman CE, Stainsby D, Wallis JP. Where does blood go? Prospective observational study of red cell transfusion in north England. *BMJ* 2002; 325: 803.

11. Avidan MS, Alcock EL, Da Fonseca J, Ponte J, Desai JB, Despotis GJ, *et al*. Comparison of structured use of routine laboratory tests or near-patient assessment with clinical judgement in the management of bleeding after cardiac surgery. *Br J Anaesth* 2004; 92: 178-86.

12. Tobin SN, Campbell DA, Boyce NW. Durability of response to a targeted intervention to modify clinician transfusion practices in a major teaching hospital. [see comment]. *Medical Journal of Australia* 2001; 174: 445-8.

13. Schramm W, von Auer F. Blood safety in the European Community (German). Bundesvereinigen fur Gesundheit (German Federal Department of Health), 2000.

14. Tamir L, Fradin Z, Fridlander M, Ashkenazi U, Zeidman A, Cohen AM, *et al*. Recombinant human erythropoietin reduces allogeneic blood transfusion requirements in patients undergoing major orthopedic surgery. *Haematologia* 2000; 30: 193-201.

Chapter 15

Haemostasis for Surgeons and Anaesthetists

Denise O'Shaughnessy FRCP FRCPath DPhil
Consultant Haematologist
Timothy Farren BSc(Hons) AIBMS
Clinical Research Fellow
Southampton University Hospital NHS Trust, Southampton, UK

"Coagulation tests are no better than the test specimen."

Introduction

The importance for surgeons of understanding the normal haemostatic mechanisms cannot be over-emphasised.

Haemostasis is a mechanism to protect the integrity of the vascular system after tissue injury and the fluidity of the blood is finely balanced between the procoagulants and the natural anticoagulants.

Excessive bleeding can be due to surgical causes, but more often is due to a derangement of haemostasis. Cardiothoracic and vascular surgery are prime examples of this.

Normal haemostasis

The *procoagulant* system of the coagulation process is a sequential activation of a number of clotting factors resulting in the formation of fibrin (Figure 1).

In vivo:

♦ The cascade is activated when tissue factor (TF), expressed on damaged cells, comes into contact with circulating factor VIIa.

♦ The combined VIIa-TF complex activates factor X and in the presence of calcium and phospholipid (from platelets), this "tenase complex" rapidly converts prothrombin (Factor II) to thrombin (Factor IIa).
♦ The initial reaction is enhanced by feedback activation.
♦ The ultimate function of thrombin is to cleave fibrinogen to fibrin and activate factor XIII to enable formation of a cross-linked stable clot [1].

In vitro:

♦ The classical waterfall hypothesis was generated to explain the prolongation of the Activated Partial Thromboplastin Time (APTT) in patients with factor XI and XII deficiency who do not usually bleed spontaneously or at surgery unless the level is very low.

The major inhibitors of the blood coagulation pathway are anti-thrombin, heparin co-factor II, protein C, protein S, and tissue factor pathway inhibitor (TFPI).

Dependence on Vitamin K

Coagulation factors II, VII, IX, X and the proteins C and S are dependent on vitamin K for their normal function. In vitamin K deficiency inactive forms are produced: proteins in vitamin K absence (PIVKAs).

Screening tests

Coagulation tests are usually performed on citrated plasma samples. The results are expressed as clotting time in seconds and compared with the mean ± 2x standard deviation of results obtained from at least 20 normal individuals, usually the laboratory staff [2,3].

Activated Partial Thromboplastin Time (APTT)

This test recalcifies citrated blood in the presence of an activator (kaolin, celite) and a source of phospholipids.

1a) Revised hypothesis of coagulation

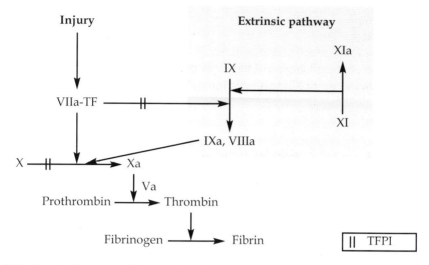

1b) Classical waterfall hypothesis of coagulation

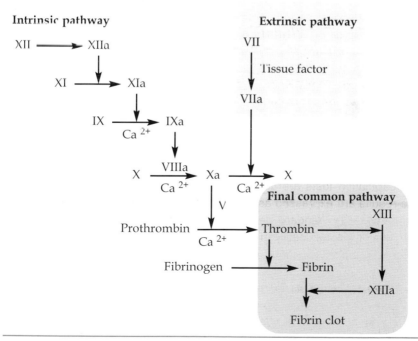

Figure 1. The classical (1b) and revised (1a) hypothesis of coagulation. TFPI = tissue factor pathway inhibitor.

- A prolonged APTT (Table 1) occurs if one or more factors in the intrinsic pathway are deficient (VIII, IX, XI, XII).
- Prolongation also occurs if there is contamination with heparin or an inhibitor such as lupus anticoagulant.
- If a mix with normal plasma does not normalise then an inhibitor to the test must be present, most likely "lupus anticoagulant", but a haematologist should advise at this point.
- The presence of heparin can be detected by adding heparinase or reptilase to the test.

Table 1. Causes of a prolonged APTT.

Common causes of a prolonged APTT

- Therapy with heparin
- Heparin contamination of sample
- Lupus anticoagulant

Less common causes of a prolonged APTT

- Haemophilia A (factor VIII deficiency)
- Haemophilia B (factor IX deficiency)
- Haemophilia C (factor XI deficiency)
- Severe Von Willebrand's disease (with a low factor VIII level)

Prothrombin Time (PT)

This test is performed by adding brain tissue thromboplastin (mainly recombinant, sometimes rabbit, but never human).

- A prolonged PT (Table 2) occurs with deficiency of factor VII in the extrinsic system.
- Prolongation also occurs with deficiencies of factors common to both systems, namely factors V, X, II and I (fibrinogen).

♦ It is particularly useful in monitoring liver damage or the effect of warfarin and other coumarin-type derivatives during anticoagulation treatment.

♦ It may also be prolonged by a lupus-like inhibitor.

Table 2. Causes of a prolonged PT.

Common causes of a prolonged PT
♦ Therapy with warfarin
♦ Obstructive jaundice or liver disease
♦ Haemorrhagic disease of the newborn (congenital or due to vitamin K deficiency)
♦ Fibrinogen deficiency
Less common causes of a prolonged PT
♦ Heparin (not if neutralised in test)
♦ Nephrotic syndrome
♦ Deficiency of factors II, VII, IX or X

International Normalised Ratio (INR)

The INR is a standardised prothrombin ratio of sample to normal control, corrected by a factor associated with the type of thromboplastin used, so that the result is universally meaningful.

Thrombin Time (TT)

Thrombin (bovine or human) is added to citrated plasma and the amount (and quality) of fibrinogen produced is measured.

♦ This test is useful for indirectly detecting hypofibrinogenaemia.

♦ It is more likely to be prolonged for spurious reasons like heparin contamination.

♦ Mild prolongation is found in renal and liver impairment.

Fibrinogen

Most automated analysers produce a derived fibrinogen result from the APTT, PT and TT.

◆ Reduced levels will occur in Disseminated Intravascular Coagulation (DIC) and hypofibrinogenaemia.
◆ To identify a dysfunctional fibrinogen, another functional test is required.

More recently developed laboratory tests

D-dimers

The breakdown products of cross-linked fibrin by plasmin generates a series of specific fragments.

Complete degradation of the clot yields a dimeric form of fragment D from adjacent fibrin monomers covalently linked. Common causes of raised D-dimers are shown in Table 3.

A wide variety of D-dimer assays are now available, namely enzyme-linked immunoabsorbant assay (ELISA), VIDAS ELISA, immunofiltration

Table 3. Raised D-dimer levels.

Common causes of raised D-dimers

◆ Venous thromboembolic disease (VTED)
◆ Thrombolytic therapy
◆ Disseminated Intravascular Coagulation (DIC)
◆ Haemorrhage or surgery
◆ Malignancy
◆ Pregnancy or intra-uterine death
◆ Liver cirrhosis and sickle cell disease

False positives may occur with

◆ Rheumatoid factor

(membrane) ELISAs, latex agglutination and whole blood agglutination. In practice, immunofiltration and immunoturbidimetric techniques combine the advantages of ELISA assays with the speed and simplicity of the first-generation latex tests and are widely used.

PFA100® system

This is a system to measure primary haemostasis *in vitro* by stimulating the *in vivo* haemodynamic conditions of platelet adhesion, activation and aggregation.

Disposable cartridges are loaded into the instrument at the start of the test. Citrated whole blood is pipetted into the cartridge and after a short incubation period, exposed to high shear before reaching a membrane coated with collagen, and either adenosine diphosphate (ADP) or epinephrine. The instrument monitors the drop in flow rate as platelets form a haemostatic plug. The closure time (CT), is normally between 80 and 180 seconds.

Although experience with the instrument is increasing, how the test should be utilised within normal laboratory practice remains to be defined. It is a potential screening tool for assessing patients with many types of platelet abnormality but it is insensitive to coagulation defects including afibrinogenemia, and haemophilia A and B.

Thrombelastography (TEG)

The TEG® analyser (Figure 2 and Table 4) measures the viscoelastic properties of whole blood producing functional profiles of haemostasis.

The TEG analyser measures the clot's physical property by the use of a cylindrical cup which holds the blood and is oscillated at a specific rate. A pin is suspended in the blood by a torsion wire and is monitored for motion. The torque of the rotating cup is transmitted to the immersed pin only after fibrin-platelet bonding has linked the cup and pin together. As the clot lyses, these bonds are broken and cup motion is diminished. The change in torque is drawn as a trace.

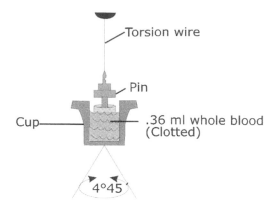

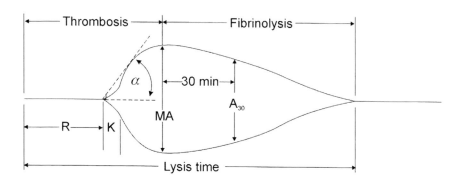

Figure 2. The Thrombelastograph trace®. The parameters are measures of global clotting function in a dynamic environment and include:
R-time = the time from the start of the trace (liquid blood) until first fibrin strand formation, a measure of clotting factors; MA = maximum amplitude of the clot, the clot strength, which in normal situations, is composed of 80% platelets and 20% fibrinogen.

Table 4. Abnormal TEG results.

Common causes of a prolonged reaction time R

- Coagulation factor deficiencies
- Excess heparin
- Severe hypofibrinogenaemia

Common causes of a reduced maximum amplitude of the trace

- Abnormal numbers or function of platelets
- Severe hypofibrinogenaemia

Activated Clotting Time (ACT)

The ACT is a test in which fresh whole blood is added to a tube containing an activator and is the test for high doses of unfractionated heparin as used in Cardio-Pulmonary Bypass (CPB).

It cannot be used in cases of heparin resistance and is likely to be inaccurate if the patient has an inhibiter-like lupus anticoagulant, in which case the Anti-Xa should be used (see below)

Anti-Xa

Heparin binds to, and enhances the activity of anti-thrombin (AT). Plasma containing heparin is incubated with AT and an excess of factor Xa. The absorbance obtained is inversely proportional to the amount of heparin in the sample.

Table 5. Measuring heparin by anti-Xa activity.

Prophylaxis LMWH	Therapy LMWH	CPB (large dose UFH)
0.2-0.4 iu/ml	0.4-1.0 iu/ml	5-8 iu/ml

When monitoring LMWH, testing should be performed 2-3 hours after the injection.

Congenital bleeding disorders detected in screening tests

Although most haemostatic defects in hospitalised patients are acquired, underlying mild hereditary disorders may only manifest in the hospital setting, such as mild haemophilia A (deficient factor VIII), mild haemophilia B (deficient factor IX), and mild haemophilia C (deficient factor XI), all of which prolong the APTT.

If patients are found to have haemophilia it is essential that a haematologist advises on best treatment which can vary from Desmopressin® (DDAVP) pre-operatively with an antifibrinolytic postoperatively, to the giving of regular doses of a recombinant replacement factor (and regular measurements of factor levels in blood) [4]. The latter may not be available in all hospitals out of hours without prior notice.

Von Willebrand's disease (VWD) is the most common inherited bleeding disorder, requiring specialised detection tests such as Von Willebrand antigen and activity, or access to a PFA100 machine. Detection is also confounded by the natural response to stress which augments the normally low Von Willebrand factor (VWF) by releasing additional product from epithelial cells. Nose bleeds and menorrhagia are the common symptoms. Most respond to intravenous or intranasal doses of DDAVP.

Hypo- or dysfibrinogenaemia will prolong the TT and reduce the fibrinogen antigen level. It is important to ask for a fibrinogen activity level, which may be considerably lower.

Acquired disorders of haemostasis in hospitalised patients

Vitamin K deficiency

Low plasma vitamin K levels, suggestive of low tissue stores, are common in intensive care patients, with or without coagulopathy.

Vitamin K absence or antagonism manifests principally as a prolongation of the PT with an increasing risk of haemorrhage.

It is therefore important to anticipate vitamin K deficiency and prevent it by supplementation in patients who are:

♦ Malnourished;
♦ Critically ill;
♦ Receiving broad spectrum antibiotics.

It is recommend that vitamin K is given to all patients at risk of, or known to have, prolonged prothrombin time. Correction, if it is going to occur, will take up to 12 hours.

Liver diseases

The synthetic function of the liver can be suppressed by hepatitis, alcohol and hepatocellular carcinoma, and results in deficiency of factors V and VII (sensitive indicators of hepatic damage) with prolongation of PT.

Factor VIII levels tend to be preserved as a result of an increased production of VWF. Hypofibrinogenaemia is also unusual.

Disseminated Intravascular Coagulation

DIC occurs when the haemostatic mechanism is triggered by:

♦ Septicaemia;
♦ Massive blood loss;
♦ Severe vessel injury or toxins (such as snake venom, amniotic fluid, pancreatic enzymes).

This may be clinically compensated and only demonstrable by laboratory tests. Decompensation will result in overt microvascular bleeding as well as microangiopathic thrombosis, as all the coagulation factors are depleted, and platelets are consumed.

The cause of DIC is not fully understood, but the best method of treatment is to treat the underlying disorder.

Cardiopulmonary bypass (CPB)

As the incidence of heart disease continues to increase, the consequent demand for coronary artery bypass grafting also increases.

Most of these procedures, together with major heart surgery on congenital defects and valvular disease, are performed on unbeating hearts supported by CPB. CPB pumps blood which is anticoagulated by large doses of heparin (3mg/kg, approximately 30,000 units) through an extracorporeal circuit with an oxygenator.

The patient's clotting is measured by the ACT and residual heparin is reversed by protamine at the end of surgery. This process:

♦ activates fibrinolysis; and
♦ disturbs platelet function.

Bleeding usually manifests postoperatively, after protamine reversal of heparin, and is shed into the mediastinal and pleural drains. If the patient is on oral anticoagulation (warfarin) that has not been reversed completely, or is on aspirin or clopidrogel therapy, there is an expectation of greater bleeding. Critical rates of blood loss are shown in Table 6.

Table 6. Critical rates of blood loss.

♦ 500mls in the first hour
♦ 800mls at 2 hours
♦ 900mls at 3 hours
♦ 1000mls at 4 hours
♦ 1200mls by 5 hours

Managing postoperative bleeding

The Mount Sinai group were the first to publish an algorithm to manage bleeding in the cardiac setting. The measurements used were partly TEG-based (celite, with and without heparinase), in conjunction with a platelet count and fibrinogen concentration from the laboratory.

- ♦ If the R-value in the non-heparinase sample was greater than twice that found in the heparinase sample, then the patient was given supplementary protamine.
- ♦ If the platelet count was <100,000 and the MA was <45mm, then platelets were administered.
- ♦ Fresh frozen plasma (FFP) was given if the celite activated R-value, ten minutes post-protamine administration, was >20mm.
- ♦ Low fibrinogen was treated with cryoprecipitate.
- ♦ Epsilon aminocaproic acid (Amicar) was given in the event of excess lysis.

Using this protocol they showed significant reductions in the use of haemostatic products compared with their more conventional transfusion protocol.

- ♦ The proportion of patients receiving FFP was four of 53 in the TEG group compared with 16 of 52 in the control group (p<0.002).
- ♦ Patients receiving platelets were seven of 53 in the TEG group compared with 15 of 52 in the control group (p<0.05)

Since then hospitals such as Harefield, Southampton and Oxford in the UK have modified this protocol and reported a similar reduction in the use of blood and blood products [5].

Conclusions

Coagulation tests are no better than the test specimen. The presence of heparin, which can contaminate blood samples taken from central venous or arterial lines, commonly results in abnormal test results, affecting the APTT and TT particularly. Faulty collection of the specimen may also lead to partial clotting and serum being tested instead of plasma. If the laboratory results do not fit the clinical picture, it is always safest to repeat the test, being more careful to eliminate these problems.

Key Summary

◆ Excessive bleeding can be due to surgical causes, but more often is due to a derangement of haemostasis.

◆ Conventional coagulation tests are performed on centrifuged citrated samples and therefore, can rarely be performed in a hurry.

◆ Of the newer tests, the TEG is most suited to provide accurate data in minimum time.

◆ Use of the TEG in protocols has been proven to reduce blood usage.

References

1. *Disorders of haemostasis and thrombosis, a clinical guide.* Goodnight SH, Hathaway WE, Eds. McGraw-Hill, 2001.
2. *Practical Haemostasis.* O'Shaughnessy DF, Makris M, Lillicrap D, Eds. Blackwell Science, Oxford, 2004.
3. *A manual of clotting disorders.* Kroll M. Blackwell Science, Oxford, 2001.
4. Joseph JE. Inherited and acquired coagulation disorders. In: *Practical Transfusion Medicine.* Murphy M, Pamphillon D. Eds. Blackwell Science, Oxford, 2001; 125-138.
5. Von Kier S, Smith A. Haemostatic Product Transfusion and Adverse outcomes, focus on near patient testing to reduce transfusion need. *Journal of Cardiothoracic and Vascular Anaesthesia* 2000; 14(3) supp 1.

Web sites

1. www.transfusion.org.uk
2. www.bcshguidelines.com

Chapter 16

Transfusion Triggers in Medical Patients with Chronic Anaemia

Clare Taylor MB BS PhD FRCP MRCPath

Consultant in General Haematology and Transfusion Medicine,
Royal Free Hospital, London and National Blood Service, North London, UK &
Honorary Senior Lecturer, Royal Free and University College Medical School, London, UK

"Although 40-50% of blood transfusions are given to support elective and emergency surgery this proportion is declining as blood conservation strategies are introduced. There are however, several approaches that can reduce inappropriate use of blood in medicine and haemato-oncology."

Introduction

Management of medical causes of anaemia is often conceptually very different from the management of surgical anaemia.

♦ Surgical anaemia is often caused by acute blood loss, whether predicted or unpredicted, whereas medical patients may have no blood loss or low-grade chronic bleeding.

♦ Surgical patients generally have a normal bone marrow with a potentially normal response to anaemia. Exceptions may be surgical oncology patients and those with severe inflammatory disease, and temporary (acute) anaemia of chronic disease (ACD) that may follow major surgery and trauma in some patients. Medical patients much more frequently have blunted erythropoietic responses, either due to ACD, with ineffective erythropoiesis, or due to the effect of drugs, or disease on the marrow.

♦ The duration of anaemia in surgical patients is generally short, with the haemoglobin (Hb) expected to rise unless there is further blood loss, while medical cases may expect to remain affected for months or permanently, and the anaemia will worsen without intervention.

- A Hb level which is acceptable transiently in a postoperative patient is often too low for a medical patient in the longer-term.
- In surgical patients the transfusion trigger is often the lowest tolerable level of anaemia, taking into account co-morbidities, knowing that it is for a short time. In medical patients one is aiming at a Hb which achieves the maximum benefit, not just physiologically, but in terms of activity levels and general well being, taking a longer-term view.

However, both haematinic deficiency and anaemia of chronic disease may contribute to anaemia in anyone and must be considered and looked for in all anaemic patients, medical or surgical.

This chapter will cover:

- Solid tumour patients on chemotherapy and radiotherapy.
- Patients with haematological malignancies.
- Transfusion-dependent myelodysplasia.
- Anaemia of chronic disease.
- Nutritional anaemias.
- Haemoglobinopathies.

General considerations in anaemic medical patients

Anaemia in medical patients is usually multifactorial and the possible impact of the following must be taken into consideration when investigating and managing them:

- Bone marrow function.
- Possible chronic blood loss and iron depletion/deficiency.
- Coagulopathy exacerbating blood loss.
- Other haematinic deficiency.
- ACD component.
- Current and planned therapy for underlying disease.
- Expected duration of anaemia.
- Severity of symptoms of fatigue and anaemia.
- Impact of co-morbidities on effect of anaemia.

- ◆ Impact of anaemia on quality of life.
- ◆ Impact of Hb on outcome of therapy.
- ◆ Potential to recover red cell mass without transfusion.
- ◆ Logistics of long-term transfusion and transfusion dependency.
- ◆ Potential role of erythropoietin therapy.
- ◆ Development of iron overload.
- ◆ Tolerance of iron therapy.

Cancer patients

The causes of anaemia in these patients may include:

- ◆ Chemotherapy and/or radiotherapy.
- ◆ Tumour infiltration of bone marrow.
- ◆ Anaemia of chronic disease.
- ◆ Haematinic deficiency.
- ◆ Bleeding and coagulopathy.
- ◆ Haemolysis.
- ◆ Decreased erythropoietin production.
- ◆ Decreased responsiveness to erythropoietin.

Practicalities

Patients may become iron deficient due to chronic blood loss directly from the tumour. This may not be easy to diagnose; ferritin is an acute phase protein and may be elevated in the presence of malignancy as well as by ACD. Iron and iron-binding capacity can also be difficult to interpret in this situation. A bone marrow aspirate will be informative about iron stores, but the marrow's histological appearance may not represent bio-available iron. An estimate of hypochromic red cells [1] is helpful and is available from most automated red cell analysers. Normal individuals have <2.5% hypochromic red cells while a figure of >10% suggests functional iron deficiency. Patients found to be iron deficient should be treated with oral ferrous sulphate 200mg tds (or equivalent) taken with ascorbic acid or citrus fruit juice to increase absorption. If this is poorly tolerated, as is often the case, intravenous (IV) iron sucrose is safe, effective and well tolerated and can be given in doses of 200mg at a time until iron repletion is achieved (calculated using the manufacturer's algorithm). The ability to respond depends on the state of the bone marrow, and will be reduced in those with extensive metastatic disease or who are hypoplastic following therapy.

Since anaemia is likely to be long-term with no chance of correction without transfusion, it is not appropriate for the transfusion trigger to be at the lowest physiologically acceptable level. Other considerations must be taken into account, such as fatigue, symptoms, activity level and general well being. A suitable target is 90-100g/L, but this may need to be higher in some patients. Quality of life (QOL) data suggests that there is a continuing correlation with increase in QOL as Hb rises to 100-110g/L and higher [2]. This is important in patients suffering from malignancies who are facing long periods of potential debility exacerbated by anaemia.

Data from head and neck cancer and also in cervical cancer patients demonstrate that Hb level during their radiotherapy influences outcome of treatment, relapse rates and survival: an Hb of >120g/L during radiotherapy is associated with an improved outcome [3]. Similar data are now becoming available relating to chemotherapy. The method of raising the Hb is not important.

Erythropoietin (EPO) has been shown to raise Hb in anaemia during and following chemotherapy in a number of solid tumours. Anaemia due to cis-platinum based regimens is particularly likely to respond, as are patients with an element of renal dysfunction, because endogenous EPO levels are lower. Patients with extensive marrow infiltration are unlikely to respond. Simultaneous iron therapy is necessary in most patients as the response is frequently limited by a shortage of bio-available iron. Use of EPO may reduce the need for blood transfusion, or increase the transfusion interval and a few patients may become transfusion-independent. Longer-acting preparations are now becoming available which simplifies administration, though costs remain high [4].

EPO is well tolerated with virtually no side effects. Pure red cell aplasia (PRCA) is a rare but serious complication of EPO administration. It has, however, only been reported after long-term use in renal patients, but not in cancer patients [5]. Suitable dosing schedules are 150mg/kg three times a week, or 40,000 IU weekly. The dose can then be adjusted up or down according to the response, which may take four weeks or more.

Haematological malignancies

These include acute leukaemias, lymphomas and chronic lymphocytic leukaemia (CLL) and myeloma.

♦ The biggest single cause of anaemia is chemotherapy, producing a predictable, cyclical anaemia with each course of therapy and almost invariably requiring repeated blood transfusion.

♦ As with solid tumours, for the sake of symptoms, QOL and the expected duration of treatment, the transfusion trigger should be no lower than 90g/L.

♦ Haematinic deficiency is possible, especially iron deficiency due to chronic blood loss, or folate deficiency due to haemolytic complications and poor dietary intake.

♦ A significant bleeding diathesis is common in this group of patients, and most frequently arises from thrombocytopenia. The presence of a paraprotein is likely to interfere with coagulation factors causing prolonged prothrombin time (PT), activated partial thromboplastin time (APTT) and thrombin time (TT). Liver dysfunction due to drugs, sepsis or disease may also play a part. Some patients may require as much as 1-2 units of blood per day to keep up with losses into the gut and tissues. In such patients platelet counts must be kept >30 x 10^9/L, rather than the usual trigger of 10 x 10^9/L for prophylaxis. Platelet increments must be documented at one hour or 24 hours post-transfusion. Platelet refractoriness (eg. increase of <5 x 10^9/L at 24 hours) should be investigated and managed with the help of the transfusion centre.

♦ ACD may contribute to anaemia and responsiveness to endogenous EPO may be poor. There is no conclusive evidence for use of EPO in acute leukaemia. Some small studies have found some response in stem cell transplantation patients, especially autologous transplants, but there was little significant impact on blood transfusion requirement.

♦ Patients with myeloma and lymphoma (including CLL) have been found to respond well to EPO with 58-85% achieving >20g/L rise in Hb above baseline [6]. This may frequently translate into a reduced or absent need for blood transfusion with a reduction in the number of hospital attendances required. In such cases EPO may prove to be cost-effective as well as preserving blood as a resource for others for whom there are no alternatives to transfusion.

♦ Iron overload becomes a problem in adults after about 50 units of blood have been transfused. On completion of treatment a course of venesection, or desferrioxamine, may be necessary.

Myelodysplastic syndromes (MDS)

♦ Anaemia is the most frequent haematological problem in this group of patients and transfusion dependency is common. Once again an appropriate trigger in such patients, who may remain transfusion-dependent for life, is 90-100g/L, and may be higher in the elderly or those with significant co-morbidities.

♦ Iron overload is a frequent problem and iron chelation may be necessary.

♦ EPO responses tend to be poor in MDS with a response rate of 16% demonstrated in a meta-analysis of 17 studies [7]. Longer treatment at higher doses may improve response rates, but is costly. Sideroblastic MDS has the best response rates. Combination therapy with granulocyte colony-stimulating factor (G-CSF) and EPO has shown some promise.

Anaemia of chronic disease (ACD)

ACD may contribute to anaemia in many situations where there is underlying malignancy, chronic inflammation, sepsis and other conditions, such as diabetes and congestive cardiac failure. It is the most frequent extra-articular manifestation of rheumatoid arthritis (RhA), occurring in between 20% to 60% of patients.

Mechanism

The underlying mechanisms remain unexplained, but there is impaired marrow utilisation of reticuloendothelial iron and a lower than expected rise in erythropoietin. The marrow also shows a blunted response to EPO. There is probably a synergistic effect of IL-1 and T cells to produce G-interferon which suppresses erythroid activity. Elevated levels of tumour necrosis factor (TNF) may also play a role.

Management

♦ Patients with ACD have an increased need for transfusion as they commence surgical or medical treatment with a lower Hb and with a poor endogenous response to anaemia.
♦ Intravenous administration of iron may improve its bio-availability and allow correction of Hb in some cases.
♦ EPO therapy has also been successful [8]; for example it can be used pre-operatively in patients with rheumatoid arthritis awaiting joint replacement.
♦ Forward planning may reduce or eliminate the need for transfusion in some of these patients.
♦ Nine percent of patients with mild CCF (NYHA class I) and 80% of those with severe disease (class IV) have anaemia defined as Hb <120g/L. Correcting anaemia with EPO/iron decreases hospitalisation and heart failure, probably by the associated 28% increase in ejection fraction [9].
♦ Recombinant human erythropoietin has proved successful in improving anaemia in patients with RhA and ACD, with nearly all patients receiving supplemental IV iron to avoid functional iron deficiency.

Nutritional anaemias

Patients with iron, B12 and folate deficiency anaemias may present with extreme anaemia (below 50g/L). When the onset has been sufficiently slow this can be well-tolerated physiologically in some patients.

Management

♦ In this instance it may not be necessary to transfuse all patients, as appropriate haematinic therapy will raise the Hb to near normal in two to four weeks.

♦ Transfusion of patients with extreme anaemia due to vitamin B12 deficiency should be undertaken with caution as it can precipitate electrolyte imbalance with cardiac arrhythmias.

♦ It is not possible to state a suitable transfusion trigger in this group of patients with nutritional anaemias and each case should be treated on the basis of thorough clinical assessment.

♦ It should be remembered that although blood transfusion will correct the anaemia it will not correct the deficiency state which must be treated fully at the same time to prevent recurrence.

Haemoglobinopathies

It is beyond the scope of this chapter to discuss the management of transfusion therapy in sickle cell anaemia and thalassaemia, but the following points are worth remembering:

♦ Folate deficiency is inevitable and will exacerbate anaemia in these haemolytic conditions unless long-term daily supplements are prescribed (5mg per day orally).

♦ Iron overload is a major and serious problem requiring active management. Iron deficiency is rare.

♦ Homozygous sickle cell disease haemoglobin (HbSS) is a low affinity Hb which delivers oxygen efficiently to the tissues in the absence of a vaso-occlusive crisis. An Hb of 80-90g/L of HbS has the equivalent oxygen carrying capacity of 120g/L of HbA. Therefore, well patients with HbSS are not strictly speaking anaemic and do not need transfusion.

♦ An Hb >100g/L (Hct 0.3) should generally be avoided in HbSS unless a full exchange has been performed as the increased blood viscosity can precipitate or exacerbate a crisis.

♦ Exchange or top-up transfusions should only be carried out under the guidance of a haematologist.

◆ Thalassaemic patients suffer anaemic symptoms at the same Hb levels as normal individuals. In order to suppress abnormal erythropoiesis and prevent development of extramedullary haemopoiesis, regular transfusion up to normal levels is required (120-130g/L).

◆ Management of thalassaemia patients should be by a multidisciplinary team led by a consultant haematologist.

Key Summary

◆ Medical anaemia requires a different approach to management than does simple surgical anaemia.

◆ The level of bone marrow function is crucial in determining the available options.

◆ The anaemia may be multifactorial and several different interventions may be necessary to correct it.

◆ Many medical anaemias may be completely or partially corrected without blood transfusion.

◆ Transfusion dependency is unavoidable in some patients and triggers should be appropriate to maintain activity levels and well being.

References

1. Macdougall IC, Cavill I, Hulme B, et al. Detection of functional iron deficiency during erythropoietin treatment: a new approach. BMJ 1992; 304 (6821): 225-6.

2. Glaspy J, Bukowski R, Steinberg D, et al. Impact of therapy with epoetin alfa on clinical outcomes in patients with nonmyeloid malignancies during cancer chemotherapy in community oncology practice. Procrit Study Group. J Clin Oncol 1997; 15 (3): 1218-34.

3. Chua DTT, Sham JST, Choy DTK. Prognostic impact of hemoglobin levels on treatment outcome in patients with nasopharyngeal carcinoma treated with sequential chemoradiotherapy or radiotherapy alone. Cancer 2004; 101(2): 307-16.

4. Gabrilove JL, Cleeland CS, Livingston RB, et al. Clinical evaluation of once-weekly dosing of epoetin alfa in chemotherapy patients: improvements in hemoglobin and

quality of life are similar to three-times-weekly dosing. *J Clin Oncol* 2001; 19 (11): 2875-82.

5.   Eckardt K-U, Casadevall N. Pure red-cell aplasia due to anti-erythropoietin antibodies. *Nephrology Dialysis Transplantation* 2003; 18(5): 865-69.

6.   Osterborg A, Brandberg Y, Molostova V, *et al*. Randomized, double-blind, placebo-controlled trial of recombinant human erythropoietin, epoetin Beta, in hematologic malignancies. *J Clin Oncol* 2002; 20 (10): 2486-94.

7.   Hellström-Lindberg E. Efficacy of erythropoietin in the myelodysplastic syndromes: a meta-analysis of 205 patients from 17 studies. *Br J Haematol* 1995; Jan, 89 (1): 67-71.

8.   Kaltwasser JP, Kessler U, Gottschalk R, *et al*. Effect of recombinant human erythropoietin and intravenous iron on anemia and disease activity in rheumatoid arthritis. *J Rheumatol* 2001; 28 (11): 2430-6.

9.   Silverberg DS, Wexler D, Sheps D, *et al*. The effect of correction of mild anemia in severe, resistant congestive heart failure using subcutaneous erythropoietin and intravenous iron: a randomized controlled study. *J Am Coll Cardiol* 2001; 37 (7) 1775-80.

Chapter 17

Assisting Patients
who Refuse Transfusion

Paul M Stevenson

Chairman, Hospital Liaison Committee for Jehovah's Witnesses, Exeter, UK

"Jehovah's Witnesses in general will accept recombinant erythropoietin; such crystalloid volume expanders as saline solution and Ringer's Lactate; colloids as dextran, gelatine, hydroxyethyl starches; controlled hypotension; perfluorochemicals; and parenteral or oral iron ... Jehovah's Witnesses deeply appreciate the professional skills of the clinicians we meet."

Introduction

There was a time when it might reasonably have been assumed that a patient who refused a blood transfusion was one of Jehovah's Witnesses. That is no longer a safe assumption. A 1996 Gallup poll claimed that 89% of Canadians "would prefer an alternative to donated blood" [1] while a July 1996 Environics poll claimed that 90% of Canadians thought "everyone should be given an alternative to blood" [1]. Subsequently, variant Creutzfeldt Jakob (vCJD) raised the profile both of the disease and of its potential to be spread by blood transfusion.

Blood transfusions have become suspect to many more than Jehovah's Witnesses; to judge the scale of this disaffection, type "bloodless medicine" into Google to find about 14,500 entries, and a further 7,500 sites for "blood transfusion dangers". Manifestly, the constituency of those refusing blood transfusion is now wider than it once was. However, while polls can provide a snapshot of public opinion in a given context, there is little if any evidence that portrays a major determination by the public to avoid at all costs the use of blood or blood products in their treatment. The probability, but no more than that, is still that the patient refusing allogeneic blood is one of Jehovah's Witnesses.

Blood in the culture of Jehovah's Witnesses

There are currently about six and a half million Witnesses worldwide, with peak support of more than 16 million persons [2]. Across such a range of racial, cultural and educational backgrounds, there can be no homogenous view of medical treatment; we are individuals with our own views on surgery, homeopathy, osteopathy, Atkins and so on. Some might have individual views on the use of antibiotics or certain blood derivatives; haemodilution, haemodialysis, bypass surgery; the gender of their obstetrician; end-of-life decisions, submitting to autopsies — about all of which the Bible says nothing. In brief, the clinician is not dealing with "a Jehovah's Witness patient" and a stereotypical medical belief package, but with "a patient who is one of Jehovah's Witnesses". Recognising this difference makes for a richly enhanced relationship, and encourages co-operation rather than confrontation.

There are, however, three aspects of healthcare on which all Jehovah's Witnesses are united. One is that we do not use tobacco, nor any addictive, non-prescription drugs [3]. A second is that we do not accept termination of pregnancy, other than in very narrow circumstances [4]. The third is that we fully exercise our right to refuse treatment involving allogeneic blood or primary blood components (i.e. red cells, white cells, platelets and plasma). Understandably, we put a great deal of effort into finding clinicians who will treat us and our families without resort to blood, operating an international network of more than 1,800 hospital liaison committees (HLCs).

Witness patients' reasons for refusing transfusion are neither quixotic nor ill-informed. They view the sacredness of blood as a core Bible teaching that points to the pouring out of the blood of the Messiah in atonement for human sin (Jeremiah 31: 31; Matthew 26: 28) [5].

The first Biblical injunction against eating blood was announced through Noah: "Every moving animal that is alive may serve as food for you. As in the case of green vegetation, I do give it all to you. Only flesh with its soul - its blood - you must not eat." (Genesis 9: 3, 4).

The nation of Israel was further bound to recognize the sacredness of blood as a symbol of life itself in many specific ways: "For the soul of the flesh is in the blood, and I myself have put it upon the altar for you to make atonement for your souls, because it is the blood that makes atonement by the soul (in it). That is why I have said to the sons of Israel: 'No soul of you must eat blood and no alien resident who is residing as an alien in your midst should eat blood.'" Neither was blood to be stored, but "poured out" and covered with dust lest any person inadvertently consume it (Leviticus 17: 10-16).

The early Christian congregation debated whether these Mosaic injunctions had relevance for them and their new non-Jewish believers. The Council of Jerusalem, through its Chairman, James, made their position clear: "Hence my decision is not to trouble those from the nations who are turning to God, but to write them to abstain from things polluted by idols and from fornication and from what is strangled and from blood." (Acts 15: 19, 20). So important was this ruling that they committed it to writing, invoking God himself in the decision: "For the holy spirit and we ourselves have favored adding no further burden to you, except these necessary things, to keep abstaining from things sacrificed to idols and from blood and from things strangled and from fornication." (Acts 15:28, 29). None of these commandments to Christians to abstain from blood was ever rescinded or amended.

By referring separately to "blood" and "what is strangled" the Bible shows that blood is to be avoided both as part of one's diet, as in the case of animals killed without draining their blood, and also as "blood" itself - a popular therapy at that time, as the second-century physician Aretaeus of Cappadocia [6], noted in commenting how blood was used to treat epilepsy: "I have seen persons holding a cup below the wound of a man recently slaughtered, and drinking a draught of the blood!" The first-century naturalist, Pliny [7], also reported that human blood was used to treat this malady.

In the 18th century, Michael Faraday, a lifelong Sandemanian, proclaimed the Biblical command to abstain from blood (Acts 15: 29). John Glas [8] had argued that God's people are under obligation to obey the restriction on blood just as the first humans had to abstain from eating the fruit of the tree of the knowledge of good and bad (Genesis 2: 16, 17). Disobedience to the command regarding blood was tantamount to a rejection of the proper use of Christ's blood, namely atonement from sin. Jesus had made a similar point about fidelity much earlier: "The person faithful in what is least is faithful also in much, and the person unrighteous in least is unrighteous also in much."

It is this historical, Scriptural and cultural background, stretching back over the millennia (and which was, until the massive casualties of World War Two made blood transfusion the treatment of choice, a mainstream religious view) that some doctors feel constrained to debate, or seek to overthrow at the bedside. We find actions at such a time intrusive. We recognize that doctors have their own core values, which are just as precious to them as ours are to us, and that there is an ethical dimension to accommodate. Writing as a journalist who is also one of Jehovah's Witnesses, I accept that we may never achieve all that we seek concerning the treatment of our minors, but I am comfortable with the balanced conclusions of the Royal College of Surgeons of England (see Table 1).

Some ethical and legal considerations

As patients, we have the right both to accept and to refuse a given treatment. While the test for competency is the *ability* to understand, believe and weigh relevant information [9] (effectively to make a reasoned decision) "there is no requirement in law that a person make an objectively *reasonable* decision" [10]. In any case, it is indisputable that what is deemed "objectively reasonable" by the medical profession would vary from year to year as evidence changes. We recognise that practitioners of medicine have to acknowledge the observation *Tempora mutantur, et nos mutamur in illis*. This goes for the practice of medicine and for patients who are Jehovah's Witnesses, who must adjust their lives and their ministry to the ambient environment. But just as there are for doctors such eternal verities as *Primum non nocere*, so there are for Witnesses eternal, non-negotiable verities such as the sacredness of blood.

This ethical dilemma of divergent priorities is enlightened somewhat by the *Code of Practice for the Surgical Management of Jehovah's Witnesses*, produced by the Royal College of Surgeons of England in 1996 and revised 2002 [11]. Some points are reproduced in Table 1.

Table 1. The Code of Practice for the Surgical Management of Jehovah's Witnesses (Paragraphs 2, 3, 5, 6, 8, 9, 16). © *2002 The Royal College of Surgeons of England. Reproduced with permission. The full text can be found at:* http://www.rcseng.ac.uk/services/publications/pdf/witness.pdf.

♦ Jehovah's Witnesses have absolutely refused the transfusion of blood and primary blood components ever since these techniques became universally available. This is a deeply-held core value, and they regard a non-consensual transfusion as a gross violation.

♦ This absolute refusal may conflict with a clinician's medical and ethical responsibility for preserving life.

♦ Jehovah's Witnesses are usually well-informed both doctrinally and regarding their right to determine their own treatment. It is not a doctor's job to question these principles, but they should discuss with Jehovah's Witness patients the medical consequences of non-transfusion in the management of their specific condition.

♦ To administer blood in the face of refusal by a patient may be unlawful and lead to criminal and/or civil proceedings.

♦ The clinician should decide whether he or she is willing to accept these limitations in management and, if so, they should plan optimal care. If not, they should refuse to operate, and the patient should be referred for a further opinion.

♦ The High Court is the most appropriate forum to achieve a fair and impartial hearing when conflict arises between religious, medical and ethical opinions.

Treating emergencies and obstetrics

The difficult areas in consent are emergencies and obstetrics. To help facilitate appropriate treatment in emergencies, most Witnesses carry a signed, dated and witnessed "No-blood Card", renewed annually or biennially [11]. It states the person's reasoned view in refusing blood transfusions, and absolves clinicians and managers from legal liability. Children of Witnesses who share their parents' beliefs, but have not yet been baptised, carry an "Identity Card", also renewed frequently. Adult Witnesses have probably also completed a Health Care Advance Directive and lodged copies with, among others, their GP [12] and hospital consultants. This states not only what treatments are unacceptable, but also individual decisions on volume expanders, blood derivatives, autologous blood salvage, haemodilution and other matters; it includes an end-of-life statement ("living will"), authority for doctors to discuss treatments with the local HLC, and specific choices in pregnancy. As ever, it is essential to engage with the patient as an individual in order to establish which products and procedures are acceptable to him or her— you will find most of us well-informed and reasonably articulate.

To help patients and clinicians faced with obstetric challenges, our Hospital Information Services (HIS) in Brooklyn, New York, monitor journals and, as needed, distribute authorised reprints to HLCs worldwide. They maintain a database of over 3,000 articles related to bloodless surgery and consult with health service providers around the world in designing effective protocols for treatment. Their fully-referenced six-page folder *Clinical strategies for avoiding and controlling haemorrhage and anaemia without blood transfusion in obstetrics and gynaecology* has been widely distributed to obstetric and gynaecology departments and midwives across the United States and Canada, and beyond. A one-page state-of-the-art *Care plan for women in labour refusing a blood transfusion* has been produced in the UK in consultation with nine consultant obstetricians, three anaesthetists, and two haematologists with special expertise in haemostasis. In 2002, HIS Britain produced a 32-page booklet on the same subject, and this too has been widely welcomed.

The *Algorithm for non-blood management of postpartum haemorrhage*, produced by HIS in New York has proved invaluable [13] in outlining the general principles for obstetric/gynaecological non-blood management (Figure 1). That chart pre-supposes an in-place strategy (Table 2), for managing the birth.

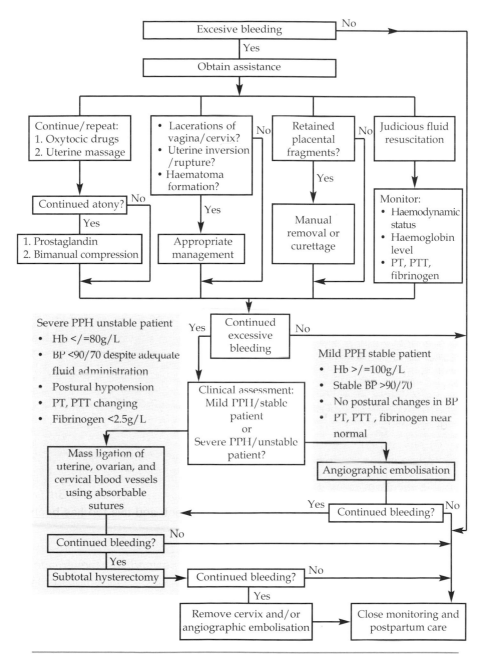

Figure 1. Algorithm for non-blood management of postpartum haemorrhage (PPH) [13].

Table 2. General principles for obstetric/gynaecological non-blood management.

♦ Prepare an individual management plan for rapid decision-making, preventing excessive blood loss by using multiple interventions.

♦ Discuss the risks and benefits of the intended procedures, getting informed consent as necessary.

♦ Ensure the availability of well-trained staff and appropriate drugs and equipment. Refer patient to another hospital if better resources are available elsewhere.

♦ Adopt an organised, team approach, seeking advice from specialists experienced in medical management without blood transfusions.

♦ Communicate the care plan to the medical and nursing staff, maintaining ongoing communication.

♦ Keep frequent, close observation for post-partum and postoperative bleeding.

♦ Recognise the clinical urgency of low-level persistent bleeding before compensatory mechanisms fail and blood pressure falls; avoid a "watch and wait" attitude.

♦ If necessary, transfer a stabilised patient to a major centre if her condition deteriorates.

To avoid and control haemorrhage and anaemia with blood transfusion in the obstetric/gynaecological ward, some general therapeutic principles are widely recognised:

♦ Thorough history-taking, physical examination, judicious laboratory investigation.

♦ Optimise the red cell mass* pre-operatively and during pregnancy.

♦ In case of severe haemorrhage, early recourse to definitive surgical measures to control blood loss is required.

♦ Use appropriate intra-operative blood conservation techniques.

♦ Restrict diagnostic phlebotomy.

◆ Normovolaemic anaemia can be well-tolerated in haemodynamically stable patients.

* Haematinics to optimise red cell mass include iron [14], folic acid [15], and Vitamin B_{12} [16].

Minors

Treatment of minors will always be contentious. Nonetheless, the standards set out by the Royal College of Surgeons in England are both workable and impartial. The HLCs poll consultants from time to time to ask them whether they are willing, in principle, and subject to their professional judgment in each case, to consider bloodless care for minors in either elective or emergency situations: having this information can speed matters up when an emergency does arise.

Jehovah's Witnesses are urged to talk to their doctor (generalist or specialist) about non-blood alternatives before the need for urgent treatment arises, particularly for pregnant women, parents with small children, and the elderly. We recommend that they commit their wishes to writing. If their clinician feels unable to treat them or their children without blood, we are usually able, through our international network, to swiftly find practitioners who can comply with their wishes. Some alternatives, like recombinant erythropoietin (EPO) with parenteral haematinics, take time to work, so we ask the friends not to postpone seeking treatment if they know they need an operation: we owe this to our doctors. A 24-hour support helpline for patients and doctors is maintained by many national offices of Jehovah's Witnesses. The local HLC can supply contact details and (if needed) immediate basic medical and legal guidance to patients and their families. It is important for doctors and managers to know that the services of HLCs are free of any charges to patients or hospitals and are available 24 hours a day, seven days a week. We are available by invitation to give presentations and show educational video material on bloodless surgery techniques and their implications to medical students, clinicians, nurses, managers, social workers, and legal representatives.

Protocols for treating patients who are Jehovah's Witnesses

Negotiations over the years have produced a very good working relationship with clinicians and hospitals in most countries where patient autonomy is recognised. This typical protocol (Table 3) was issued by the Witnesses in the US and has been adopted in many other lands, including the UK.

Table 3. Hospital protocol for treating patients who are Jehovah's Witnesses.

♦ Review non-blood medical alternatives and treat the patient without using homologous blood.

♦ Consult with colleagues experienced in non-blood alternative management at the same hospital and treat without using homologous blood.

♦ Contact local Hospital Liaison Committee for Jehovah's Witnesses for co-operative consultants at other hospitals to confer with regarding alternative care.

♦ If necessary, transfer the patient to a co-operative consultant or hospital before the patient's condition deteriorates.

♦ In a rare situation, if court assistance is deemed necessary, notify the patient, or parents, as soon as possible of such intended action. This is in harmony with natural justice and enables the court to hear both sides, including alternative non-blood medical management of the case, so as to weigh all the factors before reaching a decision.

Conclusions

Most of Jehovah's Witnesses have addressed themselves to the implications of their beliefs and have completed a Health Care Advance Directive outlining their informed decisions on matters to do with blood transfusions.

Jehovah's Witnesses in general will accept recombinant EPO; such crystalloid volume expanders as saline solution and Ringer's Lactate; colloids as dextran, gelatine, hydroxyethyl starches; controlled hypotension; perfluorochemicals; and parenteral or oral iron.

Jehovah's Witnesses will not accept transfusion of red cells, white cells, platelets or plasma; or pre-operative collection, storage and re-infusion of autologous blood.

Each patient who is one of Jehovah's Witnesses will make a subjective informed choice concerning intra-operative and postoperative blood salvage; blood derivatives such as immunoglobulins, clotting factors, growth hormones, and other proteins; haemodilution; haemodialysis and other techniques involving extra-corporeal circulation.

Jehovah's Witnesses deeply appreciate the professional skills of the clinicians we meet. We understand the dilemmas that our exercise of patient autonomy may cause them. We work very hard to co-operate with medical staff, to keep ourselves informed about medical developments involving blood, and to research alternatives and transfusion-avoidance strategies as they become available. Our culture is established, our beliefs sincere and thoroughly founded, and in all aspects of our lives our determination is firm to respect the sacredness of blood.

Key Summary

◆ There is no stereotypical Jehovah's Witness patient.

◆ Their culture concerning blood is traced over 4,000 years.

◆ They have established procedures and protocols for treating emergencies, minors, and obstetrics without allogeneic blood.

◆ They maintain a 24-hour support helpline for patients and doctors.

◆ Hospital Liaison Committees work with Witnesses and clinicians.

◆ Hospital Information Services in New York, maintains a database of over 3,000 articles related to bloodless surgery.

References

1.   Gray C. Long before Krever's report, blood scare had changed face of medicine. *Can Med Assoc J* 13 Jan 1998; 158(1): 90.

2.   *2004 Yearbook of Jehovah's Witnesses.* Watchtower Bible & Tract Society of New York Inc.

3.   Galatians 5: 20 and Revelation 22: 15 both condemn "druggery", "pharmakia" (φαρμακια), rendered "witchcraft" in KJV from the perceived association of psychedelic drugs with occult powers.

4.   *Awake!* June 1, 1994 p. 25; The Watchtower, March 15, 1975, p.191.

5.   All Scriptures are quoted from *The New World Translation of the Holy Scriptures*, published by Jehovah's Witnesses, 1984.

6.   *The Extant Works of Aretaeus, the Cappadocian.* Edited and translated by Francis Adams. The Sydenham Society, London, 1855, page 471.

7.   *Natural History.* By Pliny, XXVIII. ii. 4, the Loeb Classical Library, Vol. VIII, p.5. Harvard University Press, Cambridge, MA.

8.   *A Plain and Full Account of the Christian Practices Observed by the Church in St Martin's-le-grand, London, and other Churches in Fellowship with them.* By Samuel Pike, 1766 (London), p.28.

9.   *Re C (Refusal of Medical Treatment)* [1994] 1 FLR 31, approved in numerous cases (see for example *Re MB* (Medical Treatment) [1997] 8 Med LR 217 (CA); *St George's Healthcare NHS Trust v S* [1998] 3 All ER 673; (1998) 44 BMLR 160 (CA)) and carried over (with the addition of the ability to communicate) into the Mental Capacity Bill (2004), clause 3(i).

10. Grainger B, Margolese E, Partington E. Legal and ethical considerations in blood transfusion. *CMAJ* 1997; 156 (11 suppl): S1.

11. The BMA has recommended renewal of such documents no less frequently than every five years. *Medical Ethics Today*. BMA 1993; 6: 3.3.1.

12. As recommended in *Advance Statements About Medical Treatment*. BMA 1995; 9.1.

13. *Algorithm for non-blood management of postpartum haemorrhage*. Hospital Information Services (HIS), Brooklyn, New York.

14. Hallak M, Sharon AS Diukman R, *et al*. Supplementing iron intravenously in pregnancy. A way to avoid blood transfusions. *J Reprod Med* 1997; 42(2): 99-103.

15. Pronai W, Iiegler-Keil M, Silberbauer K, *et al*. Folic acid supplementation improves erythropoietin response. *Nephron* 1995; 71(4): 395-400.

16. Carrett NG, Ditto A, Guidoni CG. Vitamin B12 levels in pregnancy influence erythropoietin response to anemia. *Eur J Obstet Gynecol Reprod Biol* 1998; 80(1): 63.

Chapter 18

Consent and Refusal: The Competent Adult

Sheila AM McLean LLB M Litt PhD LLD (Abertay, Dundee), LLD (Edinburgh)
FRSE FRCGP FRCP(Edin) FRSA
International Bar Association Professor of Law and Ethics in Medicine,
Director, Institute of Law and Ethics in Medicine,
University of Glasgow, Glasgow, UK

"Assuming adequate disclosure of information, and that the patient is competent, it is now clear that doctors must respect the individual's decision, no matter how hard it is for them."

Introduction

Any medical treatment performed without consent is unlawful [1-3]. However, this simple statement disguises a rather more complex situation which is worth exploring briefly, before moving to the specific issue of blood transfusion. Two matters must be discussed: first, is the question of the *basis* on which a decision is made by a patient (which may of course be to refuse the recommended treatment, or select an alternative); second, is the *competence* or *capacity* of the individual to make such a choice. These very important issues will be considered in turn.

Information disclosure

Decisions made by patients in respect of treatment are usually conceptualised as an exercise in patient autonomy or self-determination. As Lord Donaldson has said:

The patient's interest consists of his right to self-determination - his right to live his own life how he wishes, even if it will damage his health or lead to his premature death. [4]

Generally, self-determination is predicated on the patient being in possession of relevant information, in order to make an informed choice. Of course, not all patients want to receive information, and in such cases their clear refusal to receive it can be construed as an autonomous act worthy of respect. However, the default position is that the clinician must be able and prepared to provide information about risks, benefits and alternatives to any patient. The law does not require that every available piece of information is made available to the patient, although a failure to provide it may result in allegations of assault (battery or trespass to the person). Rather, the law requires the doctor to disclose such risks as a responsible body of medical opinion would have disclosed - the so-called *Bolam Test* [5]. Although this test has been reconsidered, and apparently weakened, in the case of *Bolitho v City and Hackney Health Authority* [6], it remains a powerful influence on the law. In the later case, the court reaffirmed its right to decide that even a responsible body of medical opinion could be wrong, although it did say that "it will very seldom be right for a judge to reach the conclusion that views genuinely held by a competent medical expert are unreasonable." [7] This caveat has led some commentators to question just how far from the Bolam Test the law has actually moved [2,8].

Equally, the clinician will be required to disclose risks which are significant to the patient [9] (albeit that this may be decided on an objective rather than a subjective basis; that is what the reasonable patient would regard as significant). Perhaps surprisingly, there is no legal authority which requires the doctor to tell a patient all known risks even when asked a direct question [10].

UK courts have, however, held that, once a patient has been advised in broad terms of the nature of the procedure, the only possible action for patients claiming they have been given insufficient information about treatment will be that of negligence, rather than assault or battery [11]. Briefly, this entails that the claimant/pursuer has to show:

- There was a duty of care.
- That the duty was breached.
- That the breach caused the harm complained of.

This is not an easy set of hurdles for an aggrieved patient to scale. Although an offer to treat is sufficient to establish the legal duty of care, more problematic is establishing that the duty has been breached.

In this area, the Bolam Test has had an extensive - some would say insidious - impact. The question of breach of duty will primarily be judged against what a responsible body of medical opinion regards as appropriate behaviour; even where there are other responsible bodies who would disagree, and even where the "responsible body" is small in numbers [12]. Assuming that the patient can get this far, however, arguably an even greater barrier is established by the need to prove the link between a breach of duty and the harm allegedly caused by it (in law, this is known as the element of causation). This is particularly problematic where the allegation is that it was a failure to provide information that caused the harm. Courts are unsurprisingly unwilling to find for the patient where there is the risk that they are relying on the benefit of hindsight. Thus, it will not be enough for patient A to say that they would not have accepted treatment X if they had been told of the risks associated with it; the patient has to *prove* that this is the case. This is, fairly obviously, a very difficult thing to do, and courts have traditionally been reluctant to find for the patient unless an objective test (that is, what the reasonable patient would have chosen) can be satisfied.

Competence/capacity

There is a *prima facie*, but rebuttable presumption in law that an adult person is competent; that is, that they have the capacity to make binding decisions. This presumption is robust, and not easily defeated. In one case, for example, a man diagnosed as suffering from paranoid schizophrenia was held to be competent to refuse treatment that was thought to be life-saving [13]. Doctors should, therefore, be wary of assuming incompetence. The implication of this is that patients are entitled to the provision of adequate information and that, where they have "understood and retained the relevant treatment information" [14] and believed it, then their decision - however apparently rational or irrational - should be respected. The validity of a decision, therefore, is not based on how other people regard it, but rather on whether or not the individual making it has understood, retained and believed the information disclosed.

Although space does not permit in-depth consideration of those who are legally incompetent to make decisions, some attention must nonetheless be paid to them, not least because one of the major cases where competence was found to be absent relates to a refusal of blood transfusion. In the case of *Re T* [15], a young woman rejected a blood transfusion. She had been brought up as a Jehovah's Witness, although she was no longer practising that religious faith. It emerged that her mother (a devout Jehovah's Witness) had spent some time with her before she rejected the treatment. In finding Ms T's decision not to be legally binding, the court held that her competence to decide had been vitiated by the undue influence of her mother.

It must also be made clear that when adults are not competent to make decisions, their relatives have no right to decide for them. Although it might be tempting to assume that this is a legitimate way around a given problem, it is not legally the case. Although, as will be seen in the following chapter, parents can make decisions on behalf of their incompetent children, no such power vests when the patient is an adult. The law in this area has been recently clarified in Scotland, as a result of the passing of the Adults with Incapacity (Scotland) Act 2000, and seems likely to be clarified in England and Wales should the draft Mental Incapacity Bill 2003 become law. In Scotland, certain designated individuals are authorised to offer consent on behalf of an incompetent adult where the treatment is likely to be of benefit to the individual. In England and Wales, the test to be used would be that of "best interests". Additionally, the relevant Mental Health Acts specify circumstances in which others may decide for patients. Space does not permit full consideration of these exceptions here, but they can be found in the Mental Health Acts 1959 and 1983 (England and Wales) and the Mental Health (Scotland) Acts 1960 and 1984.

Refusal of consent

Religious grounds

In terms of blood transfusion, one of the most significant issues is likely to relate to refusal rather than acceptance of treatment. Most commonly, refusal will be based on religious faith, and most specifically in the case of Jehovah's Witnesses (JWs) (See also Chapter 17). There may, of course, be other reasons to refuse blood and blood products, and these will be considered below. However, most case law has centred on Jehovah's Witnesses.

JWs base their rejection of blood and blood products on a controversial interpretation of certain biblical passages: "Only flesh with its soul - its blood - you must not eat"[16] and "Keep abstaining from .... blood and from things strangled ...."[17]. JWs take these passages to amount to a prohibition on receiving blood and blood products, and - in terms of the European Convention on Human Rights incorporated into UK law by the Human Rights Act 1998 - freedom to act on religious beliefs is generally protected. A certain element of discretion is available to JWs in relation to "components such as albumin, immune globulins, and hemophiliac preparations" [18], but they claim a right to "choose nonblood medical management."[19] Importantly, as Levy points out, a "physician's familiarity with nonblood alternatives"[20] will be an important constituent of a clinician's willingness to respect such choices. Equally, it will be important that physicians are aware in these cases of alternative blood-based treatments which may be acceptable to JWs. The guide, *Family Care and Medical Management of Jehovah's Witnesses*, for example, makes it clear that:

> *Autotransfusion is acceptable to many of Jehovah's Witnesses (this being a matter of conscience) when the equipment is arranged in a closed circuit that is constantly linked to the patient's circulatory system and there is no storage of the patient's blood.*[18,21]

A series of US cases has seen courts unwilling to intervene in a competent refusal of blood transfusion [22], and may be persuasive on UK courts, particularly in light of the terms of the Human Rights Act. In addition, the fact that JWs routinely carry cards making their rejection of blood and blood products absolutely clear means that they are effectively carrying an advance directive which should - when applicable to the relevant circumstances - be respected by treating doctors. Failure to do so could result in successful legal action, as was shown in the Canadian case of *Malette v Shulman* [23]. In this case, a woman suffered grave injuries in a road traffic accident. On admission to hospital, it was discovered that she carried a JW refusal of blood card. This information was known to the treating doctor, who nonetheless proceeded to transfuse her, believing that this was the only way to save her life. In subsequent litigation she was awarded damages against the doctor.

It can be logically derived from this that a contemporaneous refusal of transfusion should also be respected, irrespective of the likely or foreseeable consequences. Sadly, at least in some situations, this has not always been accepted by physicians or by the law. Specifically in respect of pregnant women, decisions to refuse treatment - particularly in the management of labour - have in the past been rejected by courts both in the UK and in the US, on a variety of grounds, such as the importance of salvaging the foetus, or doubts about the competence of the women concerned [24]. Legal opinion is moving towards accepting the validity of women's decisions, but the fact that they were once subject to relatively regular challenge shows the extent to which it is necessary to emphasise the importance of self-determination in healthcare decisions, as in other areas of life.

Assuming adequate disclosure of information, and that the patient is competent, it is now clear that doctors must respect the individual's decision, no matter how hard it is for them. Although not a blood transfusion case, this was recently restated very firmly in the case of *Ms B v An NHS Trust* [25]. In this case, a ventilator-dependent woman requested discontinuation of the treatment, even although she was aware that this would result in her death. Her doctors believed that an alternative was available that might save her life, even though she would survive as a quadriplegic. Ms B refused to contemplate this option. The court upheld her decision, and - in an unusual move - awarded her a small sum in damages, reinforcing the fact that continued treatment in the face of a clear, competent refusal of it, amounts to an assault on the patient.

Non-religious grounds

It has already been suggested that religious faith is not the only reason for people to refuse blood transfusion. Some people will simply refuse to accept treatment at all, and - as we have seen - that is their right. However, recent understanding of the risk of infection with conditions such as human immunodeficiency virus (HIV), hepatitis C and variant Creutzfeldt Jakob disease (vCJD) may have given many people additional pause for thought. This risk was noted some years ago in a Scottish Office Report, which noted that:

Blood transfusion has a high public profile due to concerns about risks of HIV transmission and, more recently, Hepatitis C. There are alternatives to some blood products, suitable for some patients. The evidence about safety and efficacy of both alternatives and blood products is often inadequate. In many clinical cases, a simpler and safer option may be to avoid or reduce the use of blood. [26]

Yet just one year earlier, Sirchia *et al* [27], concluded from their own research that "the high use of whole blood rather than red cell concentrates in the hospitals of Great Britain .... was surprising." They also noted that "in hospitals where whole blood was not used, red cell concentrates and plasma were often used together, effectively reconstituting whole blood."

That there are risks in blood transfusion and the use of blood products can scarcely be doubted. Indeed, in December 2003 it was reported that "(a) UK patient who died from vCJD may be the first in the world to have caught the illness from a blood transfusion."[28] Patients' concern about the possibility of transmission of disease cannot be discounted, and mandates careful consideration of, and education in, alternative strategies. Both attending physicians and producers of blood products may find themselves liable to litigation; in the case of the physician under the law of negligence, and in the case of suppliers, under other legislative provision.

In the UK, for example, blood is now clearly established as a product for legal purposes, and those supplying it will be subject to what is known as a strict liability regime [29]. Unlike the situation of negligence, this means that suppliers will be subject to the terms of the Consumer Protection Act 1987, which does not require evidence of the fault which lies at the heart of the negligence action. Although certain defences are available to suppliers and producers of products, in the case of *A and Others v*

National Blood Authority [29], liability for transmission of hepatitis C was established against those who supplied the blood. Increasingly, the fact that liability can more easily be established under a strict liability regime, may encourage attempts to identify the source of the infection in order to claim damages. In the case of *AB v Glasgow and West of Scotland Blood Transfusion Service* [30], for example, an attempt was made to force disclosure of the name and address of a blood donor from whom the applicant had received HIV-infected blood, in order to seek compensation. Although the action failed, with the judge declaring "it seems to me to be impossible to hold that such a pecuniary interest should prevail over a material risk to the sufficiency of the national supply of blood for purposes of transfusion"[31], the mere fact that it was raised is cause for concern.

Conclusions

It is central to the law of medical treatment that an individual is presumed competent to make binding decisions about their healthcare management. This includes the right to make irrational or apparently inexplicable decisions. Equally, the law expects doctors to disclose the risks, benefits and alternatives to recommended therapy. In the case of blood transfusion, this may reasonably be taken to include alternatives to blood and blood products where such are available. Respect for individual autonomy also requires that physicians respect decisions taken on personal or religious grounds, even when they appear to be counter-intuitive or just downright "wrong". Doctors who fail to respect these decisions may find themselves in extreme circumstances liable in assault (battery or trespass against the person), or, more likely, in negligence. This is true whether or not the decision is contemporaneous or is made in the form of an applicable advance directive or statement. Only in cases of emergency, where the patient's wishes are not known, or in terms of the relevant legislation on mental illness or incapacity, can consent be dispensed with. It is not unreasonable in the current climate to imagine that increasing numbers of patients will seek to avoid transfusion with blood from third parties. Arguably, this mandates thorough consideration of, and research into, alternatives. The practice of medicine then becomes safer both for doctor and for patient.

Key Summary

◆ Competent adult patients have the right to accept or reject medical treatment, even if it is life-saving.

◆ Patient choice should usually be based on the provision of adequate information, which should take account of significant risks.

◆ A contemporaneous or advance refusal of treatment should be respected. In the case of the latter, the advance statement should be applicable in the circumstances.

◆ The Human Rights Act 1998 guarantees the right to act on religious beliefs, which is especially relevant in the case of Jehovah's Witnesses.

◆ Mentally disabled or mentally ill patients should not be assumed to lack competence.

◆ Relatives of an adult have no legal right to consent to or refuse treatment on their behalf. Rules for treating incompetent adults may be found in common law or various statutes.

◆ New risks from the use of blood and blood products are increasingly the subject of legal concern. Liability may be based on a strict liability regime rather than one based in negligence.

◆ The need to disclose alternatives may mandate knowledge of, and training in, alternatives to the use of blood and blood products.

References

1.   McLean SAM. *A Patient's Right to Know: Information Disclosure, the Doctor and the Law*. Dartmouth, Aldershot, 1989.

2.   Mason JK, McCall Smith RA, Laurie GT. *Law and Medical Ethics* (6th Ed). Butterworths, London, 2002.

3.   Brazier M. *Medicine, Patients and the Law* (3rd Ed). Penguin Books, 2003.

4. *Re T (adult: refusal of medical treatment)* 9 BMLR 46 (1992): 59.
5. *Bolam v Friern Hospital Management Committee* [1957] 2 All ER 118.
6. *Bolitho v City and Hackney Health Authority* 39 BMLR 1 (1997).
7. *Bolitho v City and Hackney Health Authority* 39 BMLR 1 (1997): 10.
8. Maclean AR. *Beyond Bolam and Bolitho.* 5 Med L International 205 (2002). (The test in some US states is arguably more patient-centred - see the case of *Canterbury v Spence* 409 US 1064 (1972). In Australia the Bolam Test was expressly rejected by the court in the case of *Rogers v Whittaker* 16 BMLR 148 (1993)).
9. *Pearce v United Bristol Healthcare NHS Trust* 48 BMLR 118 (1999).
10. *Blyth v Bloomsbury Health Authority* 4 Med L R 151 (1993).
11. *Chatterton v Gerson* 1 BMLR 80 (1981).
12. *De Freitas v O'Brien* 25 BMLR 51 (1995); *Simms v Simms and another* 71 BMLR 61 (2002).
13. *Re C (adult: refusal of treatment)* 15 BMLR 77 (1994).
14. *Re C (adult: refusal of treatment)* 15 BMLR 77 (1994): 82.
15. *Re T (adult: refusal of treatment)* 9 BMLR 46 (1993).
16. Genesis 9: 3,4.
17. Acts 15: 28,29.
18. Beliefs. In: *Family Care and Medical Management for Jehovah's Witnesses.* Watch Tower Bible and Tract Society of Pennsylvania, 1995: 4.
19. Ethics/Legal. In: *Family Care and Medical Management for Jehovah's Witnesses.* Watch Tower Bible and Tract Society of Pennsylvania, 1995: 4.
20. Levy JK. Jehovah's Witnesses, Pregnancy, and Blood Transfusions: A Paradigm for the Autonomy Rights of All Pregnant Women. *Journal of Law, Medicine and Ethics* 1999; 27: 184.
21. British Medical Association. *Medical Ethics Today.* BMJ Books, London, 2004: 88.
22. *In the Matter of Charles P. Osborne* 294 A.2d 372 (1972); *In the Matter of Patricia Dubreuil* 629 So.2d 819 (1994); *Public Health Trust of Dade County v Norma Wons* 541(1989); *St Mary's Hospital v Ramsey* 465 So.2d 666 (1985); *Norwood Hospital v Munoz* 409 Mass 116 (1991).
23. *Malette v Shulman.* 67 DLR. (4th) 321 (1990).
24. McLean SAM, Ramsey J. *Human Rights, Reproductive Freedom, Medicine and the Law. Medical Law International* 2002; 5(4): 239.
25. *Ms B v An NHS Trust* 65 BMLR 149 (2002).
26. Optimal Use of Donor Blood, The Scottish Office, 1995: 7.
27. Sirchia G, Giovanetti AM, McLelland B, Fracchia GN, Eds. *Safe and Good Use of Blood in Surgery (SANGUIS).* European Commission, EUR 15398 EN, 1994: 198.
28. http://www.news.bbc.co.uk accessed 29/01/2004.
29. *A and Others v National Blood Authority* 60 BMLR 1 (2001).
30. *AB v Glasgow and West of Scotland Blood Transfusion Service* 15 BMLR 91 (1989).
31. *AB v Glasgow and West of Scotland Blood Transfusion Service* 15 BMLR 91 (1989): 93.

Chapter 19

Treating Children

Sarah Joanne Elliston MA (Cantab), LLM, Barrister (non-practising)
Lecturer in Medical Law, University of Glasgow, Glasgow, UK

"Much of the following concerns situations that allow time for full discussion and in the case of serious disagreement their resolution through legal mechanisms. However, it is not uncommon for decisions concerning blood transfusions to need to be made swiftly if proposed treatment is to be effective."

Introduction

As discussed in the previous chapter, the general principle governing the acceptability of medical treatment in Europe is respect for the autonomous decision of the patient. This principle is usually enforced though the requirement of a legally valid consent to treatment.

Clearly babies and young children are incapable of evaluating treatment options so an alternative to the consent of the patient must be found to enable proper medical care to be given. As children develop intellectually and emotionally they will become more able to participate in considering their own treatment until at some point they will be regarded as having the legal right to make all such decisions themselves. The difficulty for any jurisdiction is deciding when and to what extent children and young people's decisions should be legally binding and concentration here will be on the British approach to such issues. Nevertheless, the issues raised will be relevant to those outside Britain, although the precise solutions adopted by other countries will vary. Britain in fact, has two jurisdictions, one being England and Wales and the other being Scotland. What follows is only a broad overview [1].

Preliminary issues

Who has parental rights?

A child's biological parents are generally the child's legal parents, unless he or she has been adopted, or the child was born as the result of methods of assisted reproduction governed by the Human Fertilisation and Embryology Act 1990.

If the parents are married either at the time of their child's conception or birth or afterwards, both will have parental responsibilities and rights and these survive divorce. If the parents have never married, only the mother automatically has parental responsibilities and rights although the father may acquire them through a voluntary parental responsibility agreement or a court order. Other people also can acquire parental responsibilities and rights by being appointed as guardians (on the death of parents) or on the order of a court. The term "parents" will be used to refer to those people having parental responsibilities and rights.

Parental rights and responsibilities

Parents are given the legal right to make decisions for their children, including whether medical treatment should proceed, in order that they may fulfil their parental responsibilities. Parental responsibilities are set out in the Children Act 1989 in England and Wales, and the Children (Scotland) Act 1995 (together referred to as the Children Acts). These responsibilities include safeguarding and promoting the child's health, welfare and development, providing direction and guidance to the child in a manner appropriate to the stage of the child's development and acting as the child's legal representative.

Involving the courts

Where disagreements cannot be resolved informally between parents, children and the healthcare team or there are other concerns about the welfare of the child, various legal routes can be pursued. By far the most common is to apply to a court to obtain an order in respect of parental rights and responsibilities under the Children Acts already referred to.

These enable courts to make orders permitting or prohibiting treatment. In reaching their decision the courts are required to have the child's welfare as the paramount consideration and not to make any order unless satisfied that doing so would be better than making none at all. They must also comply with the Human Rights Act 1998, and consequently, apply the rights and freedoms of the European Convention on Human Rights and Fundamental Freedoms. In addition, the courts must, so far as practicable, give the child the opportunity to express views and have regard to them, taking account of the child's age and maturity. This latter requirement, embedded in the Children Acts, reflects the rights provided for in international Declarations on the Rights of the Child to which the UK is a signatory. Even where children's views are not able to be regarded as decisive, they should be enabled to participate in decisions concerning them to the extent that this is possible and that they wish to do so. There is no minimum age restriction here and researchers, such as Alderson, suggest that children can be encouraged to participate from a very young age [2,3]. This approach is also endorsed as good practice for healthcare practitioners [4].

The courts also have inherent jurisdiction to make orders in relation to children, called the *parens patriae* jurisdiction. In England and Wales, as part of this, it is possible to make a child a ward of court so that no significant decision can be taken about the child without the court's permission. In Scotland, the inherent jurisdiction over children is rarely invoked due to the use of other options. Here, instead of using the Children (Scotland) Act 1995, cases may occasionally be referred to a Children's Hearing, which is not in fact a court, but has the power to make orders for compulsory measures of supervision of children where it is considered that they are likely either to suffer unnecessarily or to suffer serious impairment in their health or development, due to lack of parental care. Conditions can be attached to any order made, for example, to require parents to take a child to receive treatment.

Emergency treatment

Much of the following concerns situations that allow time for full discussion and in the case of serious disagreement, their resolution through legal mechanisms. However, it is not uncommon for decisions concerning blood transfusions to need to be made swiftly if proposed treatment is to be effective. In such circumstances, if no-one present can give a legally valid consent, the doctrine of necessity may apply to allow urgent and necessary treatment to be given which will safeguard the life or health of the child or prevent serious deterioration in the child's condition [5]. If however, consent is being refused by parents or the child, consideration will need to be given to whether such a refusal is legally binding and this situation will be discussed later.

Receiving blood

The most desirable situation is of course that all those concerned agree on the child's treatment. Unless the doctrine of necessity applies, treatment must be preceded by a legally valid consent or the treatment constitutes an assault (although this is more properly referred to in England and Wales as a trespass to the person or battery).

Babies and young children

Parents can give the necessary consent to allow treatment to proceed, unless there is a court order to the contrary. Where parents and the healthcare team agree that receiving a transfusion is in the child's best interests, such a decision is unlikely to be challenged. Only one parent's consent is in fact necessary to authorise treatment [6] but if parents disagree, legal proceedings may be commenced by the parent refusing consent.

In rare cases, parents may be so distressed that they cannot properly consider the issues or make a decision. In such cases treatment may proceed under the doctrine of necessity until the parents are able to resume their role as decision makers for their child [4]. This approach should be appealed to sparingly since it has been held that parents may have their human rights infringed if they are wrongly prevented from being involved in decisions about their children [7]. To make such a right meaningful, parents must be given enough information to be able to come to a decision. The issue of adequate information disclosure is dealt with in the previous chapter.

Older children and young people

There is no minimum age when children may be regarded as able to give a legally valid consent to treatment and, as has been suggested, children can be encouraged and enabled to participate in treatment decisions from surprisingly young ages. Nevertheless, clearly children will differ as to when they develop the ability to make treatment decisions and in their desire to take this kind of responsibility. In both jurisdictions, children under sixteen are presumed to be incompetent to make legally valid medical treatment decisions. However, if they can establish that they are competent to do so they can consent to treatment, including blood transfusions. At sixteen they are presumed to be competent and it would be for others to establish that they are not. However, the legal authority governing this position differs in both jurisdictions and will be dealt with briefly below.

England and Wales

The leading case for those under sixteen is that of *Gillick*, a case that gave rise to the term "Gillick competence" [8]. Although it concerned contraceptive advice and treatment it has been used to establish a general right of competent children to consent to medical treatment. This ability was described by Lord Scarman in *Gillick* as "The attainment of an age of sufficient discretion to enable him or her to exercise a wise choice in his or her own interests." Several factors will need to be taken into account. Kennedy and Grubb summarised these issues as follows:

> ... the child's understanding and intelligence, his chronological, mental and emotional age, intellectual development and maturity, his capacity to make up his own mind and his ability to understand fully, and to appraise, the medical advice being given, the nature, consequences and implications of the advised treatment, the potential risks to health and the emotional impact of either accepting or rejecting the advised treatment, and any moral and family questions involved. [9]

Advice on assessing children's competence is also given by the Department of Health [4].

The age of majority is eighteen. However, where young people are aged between sixteen and eighteen they are presumed to be capable of consenting to medical treatment on their own behalf. This position is set out in s8 of the Family Law Reform (Miscellaneous Provisions) Act 1969.

Once a young person is deemed to be competent to consent to treatment, either under *Gillick* or by statute, it is not necessary to obtain parental consent, and indeed, parents cannot override the child's consent to treatment. Despite this, it has been said that the courts can override even a competent young person's consent to treatment if the court considers that the treatment is not in the person's best interests [6]. However, it is hard to conceive of circumstances where a court would regard recognised treatment, such as a blood transfusion, that was proposed by medical practitioners and consented to by the young person, as not being in his or her best interests.

Scotland

Here, the position of those under sixteen is dealt with by statute, in the Age of Legal Capacity (Scotland) Act 1991, s.2(4). While in many respects similar to the approach taken in *Gillick*, the Scottish statute does not contain a requirement that the decision be in the child's best interests. It is also expressed in terms of the child being accorded "legal capacity". It has been argued that the effect of this is that neither parents nor courts can override the consent of a competent child to medical treatment although, due to lack of case law, the precise legal position is uncertain [1,16]. As in England and Wales however, it seems unlikely that a court would seek to override the consent of a competent young person to accept recognised medical treatment, such as blood transfusions. The issue of parents or courts wishing to dispute a child's decision is infinitely more likely to arise when a child is refusing treatment, and this will be discussed in more detail below.

Once people in Scotland reach the age of sixteen, for most purposes, including making treatment decisions, they are considered to be adults and hence presumed competent (Age of Legal Capacity Scotland Act 1991, ss 1 and 9). At this age their parents no longer have the legal right to make decisions for them and their decisions can only be challenged if they are deemed to be incompetent. If so, as adults, they would be dealt with in the ways discussed in the previous chapter. Young people in Scotland thus achieve adult status in respect of consenting to medical treatment two years earlier than their English and Welsh counterparts.

The position in respect of consenting to blood transfusion can thus be seen to be reasonably straightforward. More difficult however, is the situation where parents or children refuse consent.

Refusing blood

Babies and young children

England and Wales

A number of cases involving blood transfusions to young children have established that courts will override parental objections, usually based on religious beliefs, if treatment is deemed to be in the child's best interests [10,12]. Although the concept of best interests is not limited to medical matters [11], ordinarily it has been held that the decision taken must be that which represents the best medical option for the child, even where there are alternatives that the family would accept [12]. In only one reported case, this time involving a liver transplant, has parental refusal to consent to treatment with reasonable prospects of success been upheld by a court [11]. This case involved specific factors which may have influenced the court including the fact that the family ordinarily lived abroad and were themselves experienced healthcare practitioners. However, in all cases, the decision the court makes is said not to be based on the reasonableness of the parents' views but on the best interests of the child.

Scotland

The issue of parents refusing blood transfusions in Scotland has rarely come before the courts but it is expected that the same approach would be taken as that in England and Wales, although here the provisions of the

Children (Scotland) Act 1995 would generally be used. However, one case that did reach the courts illustrates the unique alternative jurisdiction of the Scottish Children's Hearing system. In *Finlayson, Applicant* a child was diagnosed as having haemophilia [13]. Aged six it was discovered that the boy had severe problems with his right knee due to chronic bleeding. His parents were concerned about the risk of their son contracting acquired immune deficiency syndrome (AIDS) as a result of blood transfusion and were reluctant to allow him to be treated with factor VIII. After contact with social services the case was referred to a Children's Hearing. The parents sought to challenge this referral in proceedings in the sheriff court. The sheriff held that although the parents were loving and concerned with the health of the child, their refusal to consent to conventional treatment constituted wilful neglect and lack of parental care likely to cause the child unnecessary suffering or serious impairment to his health or development. The sheriff reached this conclusion based on what a "reasonable person" would consider acceptable conduct. Accordingly, the grounds for referral to a Children's Hearing were established. While the outcome of that hearing was not published, again this case illustrates that courts will not permit parents' refusal of recognised medical treatment to put their children at risk of serious injury or illness.

Older children and young people

As we have seen, children can be deemed to be competent to consent to medical treatment either presumptively at sixteen or on establishing their competence to do so at an younger age. It might reasonably be assumed that having the right to consent to treatment would necessarily include the right to refuse treatment. However, in England and Wales the courts have held that the best interest of the child or young person permits refusal of consent to be overridden. The approach in Scotland appears to differ on this point.

England and Wales

In a series of cases after *Gillick*, the courts have held that either parents or a court can authorise treatment of a child or young person up to the age of eighteen [6,14,15]. Perhaps the most interesting case from the perspective of blood transfusions is that of *Re E* [15]. This case concerned a boy who was nearly sixteen when he was admitted to hospital suffering from leukaemia. The treatment involved blood transfusion which the family, including the boy, refused as Jehovah's Witnesses. The Health Authority applied to court for leave to treat the boy in such manner as they considered necessary, to include the use of blood transfusion. The trial judge held that the patient did not possess a full enough understanding of what his decision would involve to have his purported refusal respected. In doing so, he took into account the boy's need to be able to consider the likely manner of his dying and the effect this would have on his family. This approach is controversial, since it is quite clear from the judgment that the manner of his dying was never explained to him. As such it provided a novel way of denying competence, by effectively saying that a person is rendered incompetent when information is deliberately withheld. It is also quite unlike any test of competence that has been applied to adults in similar situations [16].

The judge also was concerned that views expressed by young people might reflect only a passing phase, and hence, did not command the same respect as an adult's decision which again is controversial [16]. In this case the court authorised treatment including transfusions until the boy's eighteenth birthday when he was legally able to refuse consent. He refused further transfusions and succumbed to his condition.

This and subsequent cases suggest that the courts apply a higher standard of competence to children's refusal of treatment than they do to either consent or in comparison with adults [17]. However, even if a child is judged competent, the courts have held that either parents or a court can override a child's refusal of consent, if treatment is believed to be in the child's best interests [6]. It has been suggested that this approach may be in breach of the child's human rights [10,19]. These might include breaches of rights under Article 8 to respect private and family life; under Article 9 to freedom of thought, conscience and religion; under Article 5 to liberty and security; and not to be discriminated against in the exercise of Convention rights, under Article 14. However, such issues have yet to be litigated here. In the event that a young person does refuse consent and is or may be competent to do so, legal advice should be sought.

Scotland

As noted earlier, the wording of the relevant statute in Scotland gives the child legal capacity when deemed competent. The Children (Scotland) Act 1995 further provides that parental rights are exercisable only for so long as the child lacks legal capacity. It may be that a court retains the ability to override a refusal of consent by a competent young person up to the age of sixteen, but this seems doubtful. Only one reported case has considered this issue. In *Houston, Applicant* [20] the sheriff held that a boy judged competent to consent to mental health treatment could not have his refusal of consent overridden by a parent. Nevertheless, compulsory treatment under mental health legislation enabled treatment to be given and the court did not consider whether it had the power to override refusal in the boy's best interests. The position cannot therefore be regarded as settled, although this case suggests that Scottish children have greater abilities to exercise autonomy in refusing consent to treatment than English or Welsh children. Nevertheless, due to the uncertainty of the legal position, where a competent child refuses treatment, such as blood transfusion, it would be advisable to seek legal advice.

Key Summary

◆ In an emergency, treatment may be given under the doctrine of necessity.

◆ In all other cases a legally valid consent is needed, which can be given by parents or competent children.

◆ Where parents refuse consent to treatment of an incompetent child, the courts may authorise treatment to proceed if this is in the child's best interest.

◆ Where a competent child refuses consent in England and Wales, parents or a court may authorise treatment to proceed if this is in the child's best interests.

◆ Where a competent child refuses consent in Scotland it may be that neither parents nor a court may authorise treatment to proceed but this is unsettled.

◆ If disagreements cannot be resolved informally, or there are concerns about the welfare of the child, legal advice should be sought.

◆ All children should be encouraged and enabled to participate in treatment decisions to the extent that they wish to do so.

References

1. British Medical Association. *Consent, Rights and Choices in Healthcare for Children and Young People.* British Medical Association, London, 2001.

2. Alderson P. *Young Children's Rights.* Jessica Kingsley, London, 2000.

3. Alderson P. *Choosing for Children.* Oxford University Press, Oxford, 1999.

4. Department of Health Seeking Consent: Working with Children. Department of Health, London, 2001.

5. *Re F (mental patient: sterilisation)* [1990] 2 Appeal Cases 1, HL. (This case concerned adults but would be equally applicable to children).

6. *Re W (a minor) (medical treatment)* [1992] 4 All England Law Reports 627, CA.

7. *Glass v United Kingdom* (2004) 77 Butterworths Medico-Legal Reports 120, ECHR; *W v UK* (1987) 10 European Human Rights Reports 29, ECHR.

8.   *Gillick v West Norfolk and Wisbech Area Health Authority* [1985] 3 All England Law Reports 402, HL.

9.   Kennedy I, Grubb A. *Principles of Medical Law*. Oxford University Press, Oxford, 1998 and cumulative supplements. Para 4.56.

10. *Re O (Medical treatment)* (1993) Times 19/3/93; *Camden LBC v R (a minor, blood transfusion)* [1993] Family Law Reports 757.

11. *Re T (a minor, medical treatment)* [1997] 1 All England Reports 906, CA.

12. *Re S (a minor, medical treatment)* [1993] 1 Family Law Reports 377.

13. *Finlayson, Applicant* 1989 Scottish Civil Law Reports 1989, Sh Ct.

14. *Re R (Wardship: medical treatment)* [1991] 4 All England Reports 177, CA; *Re K, W and H (minors, medical treatment)* [1993] 1 Family Law Reports 854.

15. *Re E (a minor, wardship medical treatment)* [1993] 1 Family Law Reports 386.

16. Elliston S. "If You Know What's Good for You...": A Consideration of Refusal of Consent to Medical Treatment by Children. In: *Contemporary Issues in Law, Medicine and Ethics*. McLean SAM, Ed. Dartmouth Publishing Co, Aldershot, 1996: 29-55.

17. *Re L (medical treatment, Gillick competence)* (1998) 51 Butterworths Medico-Legal Reports 137.

18. British Medical Association: The Impact of the Human Rights Act 1998 on Medical Decision-Making. British Medical Association, London, 2000.

19. Wicks E. The Right to Refuse Medical Treatment under the European Convention on Human Rights. *Medical Law Review* 2001; 9: 17-40.

20. *Houston, Applicant* 1996 Scottish Civil Law Reports 943.

Chapter 20

Mismatching Errors in the Blood Transfusion Process

Margaret O'Donovan RN PGdip MIHM

Risk Manager, Royal Free Hospital NHS Trust

Hampstead Heath, London, UK

"Safety must be recognised as a systems problem, and as a dynamic process, rather than a static characteristic."

Introduction

In transfusion medicine mismatching errors have an increased potential for patient harm because of their possible combination with blood group incompatibility [1]. Among the complications arising from blood transfusion are transfusion transmitted infections, immune complications, and incorrect blood components transfused. In the UK, the Serious Hazards of Transfusion (SHOT) data from the years 1996/7-2001/2 suggests that 41 deaths were attributed to transfusion, and another 29 deaths probably attributed to transfusion [2]. The largest category was found to be Incorrect Blood Component Transfused (IBCT), accounting for 1,711 (63.9%) of all errors reported during the period of 1996/7-2001/2 and 343/478 (71.8% for 2001/2002).

Mismatching in blood transfusion is a major concern. Guidelines and recommendations issued by major patient safety bodies place a strong emphasis on the rigid enforcement of formal procedures, policies, and training and education programmes. However, there is little guidance with regard to how enforcement could be carried out in order to minimise the likelihood of non-compliance.

Recommendations for reducing mismatching errors have involved the use of several patient identifiers, piloting of technology, active patient involvement and incident reporting systems. Additional useful manual processes include bay layout in hospitals and personal knowledge of patients by nurses. Although all of the recommendations have their place and utility, they do not systematically address underlying factors likely to affect their effectiveness.

Patient identification and the prevention of mismatching is a big concern of the major medical bodies, such as the patient safety organisations in the US, the Joint Commission for Accreditation of Healthcare Organisation (JCAHO) and the Association of Operating Room Nurses (AORN); in the UK, the Nursing and Midwifery Council (NMC). These bodies have issued a range of guidelines and recommendations, which have been reviewed. Many of the recommendations have high face-validity, even though little scientific evidence or published literature about their impact is available.

The guidelines place a strong emphasis on having procedures and policies in place, and rigidly enforcing them. There is, however, little guidance available on how to maximize procedure compliance apart from traditional approaches such as sanctions and blame, which usually do not address the underlying causes of non-compliance. In addition, there are no studies available which analyse the impact of different ways of introducing and maintaining procedures.

The replacement of permanent nurses with agency staff, including contracted external healthcare assistants, who move around frequently and do not have the opportunity to build up and maintain local knowledge, may contribute to the failure of checks for a number of reasons. These include:

- A lack of knowledge of who to contact and how to proceed in the case of absent wristbands.
- Increased time pressure due to lack of familiarity with the local environment.
- Increased communication problems due to lack of knowledge of the local work practices.
- Over-reliance on previously conducted checks by permanent staff.

Unless these underlying factors are addressed systematically, the recommendations issued by the medical bodies may fail to realize their full potential.

Misidentification - the size of the problem

Serious Hazards of Transfusion (SHOT): Annual Report 2001/2002

The Serious Hazards of Transfusion (SHOT) voluntary reporting scheme [2] was launched in November 1996, and aims to collect anonymised (for both patient and hospital) data on serious events of transfusion of blood components. Because of the annual SHOT reports, incidents in transfusion are among the better documented adverse events in the UK. The data from the Annual Report 2001/2002 are outlined below.

Incorrect Blood Component Transfused (IBCT) is defined as all episodes where a patient was transfused with a blood component or plasma product which did not meet the appropriate requirements or which was intended for another patient.

Adverse IBCT events reported during the last six years (in relation to the total number of adverse events) are shown in Table 1.

Table 1. Adverse IBCT events reported during the last six years.

	1996/ 1997	1997/ 1998	1998/ 1999	1999/ 2000	2000/ 2001	2001/ 2002	Total
IBCT	81	110	144	201	213	258	749
Total	169	196	255	293	315	343	1571

IBCT represents the largest error category.

Table 2 indicates the transfusion-related mortality/morbidity overall and due to IBCT.

Table 2. The transfusion-related mortality/morbidity due to IBCT.

	IBCT 2001/2002	IBCT 1996-2002
Death definitely attributed to transfusion	0	5
Death probably attributed to transfusion	1	2
Death possibly attributed to transfusion	3	8
Death due to underlying condition	18	74
Major morbidity	9	69
Minor or no morbidity	310	876
Outcome unstated	5	11
Total	**346**	**1045**

In the 346 cases analysed relating to IBCT in 2001/2002, 552 errors were reported in the categories outlined in Table 3.

Table 3. Errors reported in IBCT cases in 2001/2002.

Category	Errors reported (%)
Collection, administration	236 (42.7%)
Hospital blood bank	157 (28.4%)
Prescription, sampling, request	149 (26.9)
Blood centre	6 (1%)
Other	4 (1%)

Contributing factors were:

- Confusion over patients with similar names.
- Checking remote from the patient's bedside (for example, at the ward desk).
- Interruption between completion of the checking procedure and administration of the transfusion.
- Failure to note discrepancies between compatibility and donation labels.

The withdrawal of the wrong component from its storage location by porters and nurses continues to be a problem.

A contributing factor to the 33 failures of requesting the appropriate components was the failure to supply relevant clinical information on request forms and the failure of communication between hospitals when transferring patients.

Bar code technology: its role in increasing safety of blood transfusion

Turner *et al* [3] analysed 51 first units of red cell transfusions before and after the introduction of a bar coding system in a haematology outpatient clinic in the UK (1500-bed hospital). The study revealed that during the administration of blood, patients were not asked for their name in 93% of the cases, while their date of birth was not asked in 12%. In 12% of cases, the patient was not wearing a wristband, and in 100% of cases, the patient ID on the wristband was not cross-referenced with the patient-stated ID. In 90% of the cases, the special requirements on the blood pack were not cross-referenced with any requested on the prescription. All the checks were carried out at the bedside. During the collection of blood samples (30 observations), 43% of the patients were not asked for their name, while 50% were not asked for their date of birth. Ninety percent of the patients were not wearing a wristband. The results are summarised in Table 4, including the figures obtained after the introduction of the bar code system (after a one-month familiarisation period).

Table 4. Results of red cell transfusions before and after the introduction of a bar coding system in a haematology outpatient clinic in the UK.

Audit measures: blood administration	Manual (n=51)	Bar code (n=51)
Patient asked to state full name	7 (14%)	51 (100%)
Patient asked to state date of birth	45 (88%)	51 (100%)
Patient wearing an ID wristband	45 (88%)	50 (98%)
Patient wearing a red label wristband	49 (96%)	Not applicable
Patient ID on wristband cross-referenced with patient-stated ID	0 (0%)	51 (100%)
Patient's red label number on wristband checked and corrected	44 (86%)	N/A
Expiry date of blood checked	49 (96%)	51 (100%)
Special requirements on the blood pack cross-referenced with any indicated on the transfusion report form	44 (86%)	49 (96%)
Special requirements on the blood pack cross-referenced with any requested on the prescription	5 (10%)	21 (41%)

Audit measures: blood sample collection	Manual (n=30)	Bar code (n=30)
Patient asked to state full name	17 (57%)	25 (83%)
Patient asked to state date of birth	15 (50%)	25 (83%)
Patient wearing an ID wristband	3 (10%)	30 (100%)
Patient ID on wristband checked	1/3 (33%)	30 (100%)
Phlebotomist placed a red label in the medical notes	29 (97%)	N/A
Red label wristband attached to the patient	3 (10%)	N/A
Phlebotomist advised patient to retain their red label for later hospital attendance	14 (47%)	N/A
Sample tube labelled immediately	28 (93%)	N/A
Patient's DOB entered correctly on the sample tube	29 (97%)	30 (100%)
Patient's gender entered correctly on the sample tube	16 (53%)	30 (100%)

Some underlying causes reported were:

◆ Frequent distraction and interruptions while checking blood.
◆ Complexity of the activity.
◆ Lack of formal regular education and training.
◆ Human error.
◆ Perception that the procedure was not appropriate/efficient.

Bedside transfusion errors

Baele *et al* [4] assessed the frequency and nature of bedside errors in three hospitals. Over a period of 15 months, 808 patients received 3,485 units. 163 errors were detected, 13 of them major.

The results are summarised in Table 5.

Table 5. Frequency and nature of bedside errors.

Error type	No cases reported
Misidentification of patient	7 (major)
Transfusion of allogeneic unit when autologous blood was available	5 (major)
Transfusion when crossmatch was ordered	1 (major)
Misrecording	61
Mislabelling	6
Failure to document transfusion adequately	83

Unit placement errors: a potential risk factor for ABO and Rh incompatible blood transfusions

Shulman *et al* [5] investigated the incidence of unit placement errors in a large institution. Unit placement errors can be particularly hazardous in emergency situations when un-crossmatched blood is transfused. The study examined 96,581 units and found an error rate of 0.12% (112 units misplaced), with about one third of these potentially leading to ABO-incompatible transfusions if released (ABO mismatch error rate of 0.04%).

Monitoring transfusionist practices: a strategy for improving transfusion safety

Shulman *et al* [6] identified the following causes for variance from procedures:

- ◆ Insufficient knowledge because of a deficiency in orientation or training.
- ◆ Performance deficiency caused by lack of acceptance of the procedures.
- ◆ Indifference or carelessness.
- ◆ System deficits.

College of American Pathologists (CAP) Q-Probes Study on transfusion procedures

Novis *et al* [7] showed that complete adherence to optimal patient identification protocols was 62% in 660 hospitals.

Summary of the literature

There is a substantial amount of literature on errors in blood transfusion in general, and on mismatching errors specifically. The SHOT report suggests that IBCT represents the largest error category (67%). An estimate suggests that administration of wrong blood or blood to the wrong patient occurs at a rate of 1 per 12,000 units. Adherence to the official protocol for patient identification was found to be 62% in one study, and to a maximum of 14% in a second study (cross-referencing information, and checking full patient ID information appear to be particularly problematic). The studies suggest that failure to correctly identify the patient at the bedside appears to be the largest problem

(23.8% in the SHOT 2000/2001 report). Another study reported 61% of errors related to failures in bedside patient identification.

The literature also suggests that the failure of bedside identity checking is the major contributing factor to mismatching. However, it is likely that this is due to the fact that bedside identity checking is the last point of recovery, where errors will become apparent. In addition, we may expect that a large number of errors committed earlier in the process will be recovered through bedside verification, and therefore go unnoticed and unreported. We may assume that a more in-depth process analysis would reveal a larger number of errors in the earlier stages in the process, thereby decreasing the percentage of failures attributable exclusively to a failure in bedside identity checking.

Documented recommendations and procedures

The guidance provided by SHOT and the British Committee for Standards in Haematology (BCSH) is the way forward for now, until technological solutions such as bar coding and radio frequency identifation (RFiD) have been successfully piloted and tested, and are seen to be a sustainable solution within the health service.

SHOT 2001/2002 Report

There are specific recommendations in the report to avoid the wrong blood component or wrong patient errors:

♦ Formal policy, including formal identification procedure.
♦ Formal policy for bedside checks, rigidly enforced.
♦ Patients uniquely identified.
♦ Individuals responsible for prescription/request must be familiar with the patient's needs.
♦ Strict procedures for taking samples (eg. one sample at a time).
♦ Blood banks need to ensure they meet current guidelines.
♦ Formal recording of telephone requests.

BCSH guidelines

The BCSH has produced guidelines on *Administration of blood and blood components*, from which local policies and written procedures can be developed.

The following is a description of a standard transfusion procedure without bar coding technology (British Committee for Standards in Haematology and additional practices employed by the John Radcliffe Hospital Oxford):

A unique number is allocated to each patient at the time of blood sample collection for compatibility testing. The number is printed on labels on a red strip - 10 red labels with the same number per strip. One label from the strip is attached to each of the following: patient (wristband), sample tube, request form, and the descriptive section of medical notes. After crossmatching, the blood bank computer prints the red label number on the compatibility label attached to the unit of blood and the transfusion report form.

The process of patient identification before administration of each blood product is as follows:

- Patient states first name, surname, and date of birth.
- Details are checked against prescription chart, medical notes, transfusion report form, and the patient's wristband.
- Patient's hospital and red label numbers on wristband are checked against numbers on prescription chart, etc.

The patient identification before blood sample collection is as described above.

Common failures have been highlighted:

- Failure to ask patient for ID details.
- Use of secondary identifiers.
- Failure to use wristbands.
- Failure to issue a patient ID.

◆ Pre-labelling of samples.
◆ Failure to label sample before moving to the next patient.
◆ Failure to indicate special requirements.
◆ Failure to check historical patient record.
◆ Failure to provide adequate patient identification during telephone requests.

Other safety issues

Other issues include: technical aspects, care and monitoring, management and reporting of adverse events, documentation, staff responsible, training, IT, and out-of-hospital transfusion.

Reason [8] describes a long list of measures that have been commonly employed, such as selection, training, licensing and certification, skill checks, human resource management, quality monitoring and auditing, technical safety audits, unsafe acts audits, hazard management systems, procedures, checklists, rules and regulations, administrative controls, total quality management, probabilistic safety assessment, fault tree analysis, human reliability analysis, Hazard and Operability Studies (HAZOP), and Failure Modes and Effects Analysis (FMEA). Emphasis is placed however, on the following selection:

◆ Standards relating to risk management.
◆ Root cause analysis.
◆ Incident and near miss reporting.
◆ Training: crew resource management.
◆ Safety culture.
◆ Human factors engineering / human centered design.

As van der Schaaf [9] points out, without proper changes in culture, perspective and attitude towards errors, failures and their causes, introducing tools and technological solutions with the hope of a "quick fix", will probably be unsuccessful. Safety must be recognized as a systems problem, and as a dynamic process, rather than a static characteristic.

Root Cause Analysis

Root Cause Analysis (RCA) has been useful in establishing underlying factors influencing the likelihood of accidents. For this reason, it is widely adopted by investigators in various industries, eg. airline, nuclear, chemical and now in the National Health Service, in order to establish why accidents occurred, i.e. to identify the root causes underlying accidents, rather than simply describing the surface symptoms. RCA usually provides much deeper insights into why and how things went wrong than would be possible by assessing incident reports (described below). On the other hand, it is a much more labour-intensive process. RCA usually involves establishing the sequence of events that happened, and then systematically identifying the underlying factors. The US Department of Energy issued a Root Cause Analysis Guidance Document (http://tis.eh.doe.gov/techstds/standard/nst1004/nst1004.pdf) where a five-step RCA process is recommended.

1. Data Collection:

♦ Conditions immediately before, during and after the event.
♦ People involved, environmental factors, and other issues of relevance.

2. Assessment: application of a causal analysis technique, in order to establish immediate causes, and the reasons why these causes existed, until root causes are reached.
3. Corrective actions: implementation of corrective actions in order to prevent such an event or similar events from recurring.
4. Inform: filing of data in a central system.
5. Follow-up: determining whether corrective actions have been effective.

Carroll et al [10] describes an additional important insight gained through the introduction of a RCA intervention in a chemical refinery. For a three-week period, staff were trained in the application of RCA. During that period, team members became aware that the RCA learning intervention actually led to more disciplined thinking about problems and a shift towards more trust and openness. As Carroll et al states, these beneficial effects were not direct consequences of the tool (RCA) as such, but rather were due to the way the tool was put to use.

Reason [8] identifies four critical components of a safety culture:

- ♦ Reporting culture: an organisational climate where people are prepared to report errors and near misses.
- ♦ Just culture: an effective reporting system depends on how an organization handles blame and punishment. A just culture implies an atmosphere of trust in which people are encouraged to provide safety-related information, while still maintaining a clear distinction between acceptable and unacceptable behaviour.
- ♦ Flexible culture: ability for reconfiguration in the face of emergency or critical situations, for example through shifting from a hierarchical mode of operation to a flatter structure.
- ♦ Informed culture: a process or the ability to acquire and maintain knowledge about the human, technical and organisational factors determining the safety of the system as a whole.

Accessing the impact of a safety culture is difficult, since it is a dynamic process combining many interacting elements.

Incident and near miss reporting

Barach and Small [11] note that there is a long tradition in healthcare to report medical mishaps. However, they point out that current practices such as conferences on morbidity and mortality, grand rounds, and peer review all share the same shortcomings: a lack of human factors and thinking about systems; a narrow focus on individual performance to the exclusion of contributory team and larger social issues; hindsight bias; a tendency to search for errors as opposed to the myriad causes of error induction; and a lack of multidisciplinary integration into an organisational side safety culture.

Analysis of the number and types of events reported to, for example, the JCAHO or SHOT reveals clearly that the focus is on events with adverse outcomes. JCAHO reviewed only 2,085 events from 1995-2003, while

SHOT received 1,228 report forms from 1996-2001. However, SHOT additionally invited participating hospitals to report near misses, but as stated in the report of 2000/2001, disappointingly, only 452 near misses have been reported. The Agency for Healthcare Research and Quality (AHRQ) report [12] states that studies have shown only 1.5% of all adverse events result in an incident report. The American College of Surgeons estimates that incident reports generally capture 5-30% of adverse events. This shows clearly that compared to other high-risk industries, reporting of adverse events, and even more so reporting of near misses, is seriously deficient.

The use of technology in blood transfusion

There is little doubt that technology will increasingly be introduced into healthcare settings for performing various functions not only related to treatment, but also to logistics and administration. In the special case of preventing mismatch it is anticipated that technology such as bar coding may be a helpful tool. However, this does not imply that "manual" processes will disappear. In addition, it cannot be guaranteed that a potential technology will turn out to be helpful in actual practice. A technological tool is simply yet another artefact being introduced into everyday activities, and will need to be understood and designed as such. Professionals working in healthcare, such as nurses, will use the new tools to achieve their objectives, although not necessarily in the ways intended by the designers.

The introduction of technological solutions without a thorough analysis of how people will work with the technology, and a comprehensive understanding of the cultural, organisational and social dimensions of their context of use, is likely to lead to expensive failures. It is equally clear, however, that there are enormous opportunities in the healthcare sector to learn from the mistakes of traditional safety-critical industries. This will ensure that comprehensive risk management systems are implemented to minimise the likelihood of adverse events by the effective combination of technological innovations and human flexibility and ingenuity.

Conclusions

- Incorrect Blood Component Transfused (IBCT) is the largest error category.
- Wrong patient errors may occur at a rate of 1/12,000 units transfused.

Key Summary

Recommendations for safer blood transfusion:

- There is a need to provide training to people involved in risk assessment and risk management. Guidelines and recommendations relevant to incident reporting should be issued.
- Risk assessment should include the specific application context and should not rely exclusively on the assessments produced by medical device manufacturers. In particular, the establishment of the role of a systems integrator in hospitals should be considered.
- The assessment of underlying contextual factors contributing to incidents and accidents should be routinely carried out. Such an assessment can be linked to incident reporting systems.
- Pilot studies concerned with the introduction of new technology should consider the actual working practices of staff.

References

1. Linden JV, Kaplan HS. Transfusion Errors. *Transfusion Medicine Reviews* 1994; 8(3): 169-183.
2. Serious Hazards of Transfusion (SHOT). Annual Report 2001/2002.

3. Turner CL, *et al*. Barcoding Technology: its role in increasing safety of blood transfusion. *Transfusion* 2003; 43(9): 1200-9.

4. Baele PL, *et al*. Bedside transfusion errors. *Vox Sang* 1994; 66: 117-121.

5. Shulman IA, Kent D. Unit placement errors: a potential risk factor for ABO and Rh incompatible blood transfusions. *Lab Med* 1991; 22: 194-196.

6. Shulman IA, *et al*., Monitoring transfusion practices: a strategy for improving transfusion safety. *Transfusion* 1994; 34: 11-15.

7. Novis DA, *et al*. Audit of transfusion procedures in 660 hospitals. *Arch Pathol Lab Med* 2003; 27: 541-548.

8. Reason J. *Managing the Risk of Organisational Accidents*. Ashgate Publishing, 1997.

9. van der Schaaf TW. Medical applications of industrial safety science. *Quality and Safety in Health Care* 2002; 1(3): 205-6.

10. Carroll JS, *et al*. Lessons learned from non-medical industries: root cause analysis as culture change at a chemical plant. *Quality and Safety in Healthcare* (England) 2002; 11(3): 266-9.

11. Barach P, Small SD. Reporting and preventing medical mishaps: lessons from non-medical near miss reporting systems. *BMJ* 2000; 320(7237): 759-63.

12. Shojania KG, *et al*. *Making Health Care Safer: A Critical Analysis of Patient Safety Practices*. Agency for Healthcare Research and Quality publication 01- E058, 2001.

Chapter 21

Audit and Clinical Governance

Richard Lee BSc FRCP FRCPath
Consultant Haematologist
Bruce Campbell MS FRCP FRCS
Professor & Consultant Surgeon
Royal Devon & Exeter Hospital, Exeter, UK

"Even now, some practices in transfusion medicine continue to be embedded in tradition rather than evidence."

Clinical audit and governance

Clinical audit has always been part and parcel of clinicians' practice, but only in recent times has it been clearly defined and formalised. It simply means that clinicians look at what they are doing in a critical way, change their practice when there is a need, and then look again. It should result in a continuous spiral of improvement. Collecting data for audit may involve continuous monitoring, or it may take the form of episodic studies in selected areas of practice. Choosing acceptable or desirable standards of practice with which to compare audited data is a fundamental principle. These can be used to monitor and compare the performance of different clinicians or units nationally.

The idea of clinical governance was introduced to the NHS in the late 1990s [1], derived from the concept of corporate governance in business. It imposed a duty on Chief Executives of hospital Trusts to identify areas of practice which ought to be improved, and to demonstrate that action had been taken to improve them. Clinical audit therefore, came to fall under the general umbrella of governance. Introduction of governance gave clinical audit a mandate which had been lacking.

The NHS Executive has defined clinical governance as "a framework through which NHS organisations are accountable for continuously improving the quality of their services and safeguarding high standards of care by creating an environment in which excellence in clinical care will flourish" [1]. The Commission for Health Improvement (CHI) offered a further clarification describing clinical governance as "the framework through which NHS organisations and their staff are accountable for the quality of patient care, including a patient-centred approach, up-to-date clinical care, high standards and safety, and improvement in patient services and care".

The structure of clinical governance has now been built into all Trusts. Clinical governance committees have been established with the Chief Executive as the accountable officer, and the Medical Director as the lead clinician, who is responsible for ensuring that systems for clinical governance are in place and for monitoring their continued effectiveness.

The governance process

It is essentially a process of controls assurance [2] in which:

♦ "the way to do things" is defined in standard operational procedures, policies and protocols, i.e. standards;

♦ ways of measuring "the way things are being done" are introduced to indicate whether the organisation is working as intended, i.e. audit; and

♦ risks are identified and action is taken to reduce those risks, i.e. risk management.

Underlying this process are the concepts of clinical effectiveness and evidence-based practice. Clinical effectiveness means ensuring that effective interventions are introduced and ineffective interventions are discontinued. Evidence-based practice means that interventions are supported by best available evidence. It is a sobering thought that blood transfusion practice grew from the imperatives of war long before it could be subjected to rigorous scientific and clinical trial. Even now, some practices in transfusion medicine continue to be embedded in tradition rather than evidence.

Good practice

Although formal clinical governance is a recent introduction to the NHS, its principles have long been established in good medical practice. In blood transfusion, good manufacturing practice, product liability, quality control and audit of blood use have been familiar aspects of daily practice for those involved in the long blood supply chain [3a-d].

Haematologists, biomedical scientists and blood bank managers are well-accustomed to control systems that ensure analytical accuracy, and precision and quality checks are mandatory parts of standard operational procedures. Satisfactory performance in National External Quality Assurance Schemes (NEQAS) has always been a requirement for Clinical Pathology Accreditation (CPA).

Audit and safer blood transfusion

History

Audit is regarded as one of the pillars of clinical governance, but it is interesting to note that the Department of Health first recommended audit as long ago as 1951 [4] when blood transfusion as standard treatment was in its infancy. Even then it was recognised that "blood and, to a lesser extent, its derivatives, are also potentially dangerous materials" and that "since blood and its derivatives, such as plasma, can be obtained only from human volunteers their provision cannot be indefinitely increased".

The problems of transfusion hazards and inadequate supply are interlinked and are as pressing today as they were then. The recommendation by the Ministry of Health "to have the use of blood, as revealed by the register, discussed at intervals at the hospital medical staff meetings" may have sown the seeds of the idea of audit and Hospital Transfusion Committees (HTCs). However, it was in the US that guidelines for improving practice, supervised by HTCs first emerged [5]. Not until 1990, following a national review of pathology services, did officials recommend that every hospital in the UK should have a transfusion committee.

Modern practice

Two recent Health Service Circulars in 1998 [6] and 2002 [7] have focused attention on blood transfusion practice in the UK and firmly place the objective of making it safer in the hands of Trust management as part of clinical governance responsibilities. Other objectives in the programme of action include the avoidance of unnecessary use of blood, and better information to patients and the public. In all these areas progress is being made, but continued vigilance is necessary because blood transfusion will always be associated with some risk.

The blood transfusion process involves many steps, all of them prone to error. From donor-related procedures to the bedside checks, there is ample potential for human and systems failure. Examination of all of these steps with the aim of improving the outcome of the process must have a high priority in any audit programme.

Local hospital-based audits are necessary to ensure compliance with local policies and to improve practice. Comparative audit with feedback in anonymised form, is a powerful tool for detecting clinically significant variations in practice and for effecting change through peer pressure. However, national audits have greater potential for effecting change through the development of national guidelines [8] and benchmarks [9].

A national audit of the blood transfusion process in the UK [10] provided important data confirming a significant shortfall in the systems for monitoring and delivering transfusions in many hospitals. This information and the Serious Hazards of Transfusion (SHOT) scheme of haemovigilance [11] led to guidelines on blood handling and administration, and have given the initiatives for risk reduction a higher profile [7].

A national comparative audit of blood transfusion practice has recently been completed (in press), and all HTCs should be able to assess their hospital's performance against standards achieved elsewhere and take steps to remedy poor performance, where identified.

Avoiding transfusion

Various risk reduction strategies are rightly being pursued with vigour, from improved donor selection and testing procedures, to electronic crossmatching and automated systems for the transfusion process, but a strategy that deserves much greater prominence is the avoidance of transfusion. There is no better way to avoid all the risks of blood than by not having a transfusion, if it is clinically safe to do so.

Audit has shown huge variation in blood usage for common surgical operations throughout Europe [12], suggesting that inappropriate transfusion is common. Transfusion thresholds have long been debated but a recent systematic review based on ten trials suggests a restrictive strategy for blood transfusions is safe in the absence of significant bleeding and evidence of serious heart disease [13]. However, this review failed to take account of quality of life improvements, which have previously been shown to correlate with haemoglobin levels in cancer patients [14]. Therefore, other interventions, such as the use of erythropoietin (EPO), need to be considered and funded. EPO use in UK cancer patients runs at much lower levels than in most of Europe [15] and since approximately 30% of red cell transfusions are for cancer patients there is scope for blood conservation through the promotion of alternatives in this patient group. The implications for drug budgets will need to be addressed if this objective is to be met.

Guidelines

For busy clinicians at the bedside and in the operating theatre, faced with the daily dilemma to transfuse or not to transfuse, the difficulties cannot be eliminated, but they can be eased by better information, audit and education. Theoretically, guidelines are helpful in these circumstances, but they must be widely disseminated, easily accessible and appropriate to the clinical specialty. Any guidelines need to be authoritative with a very clear summary of the main recommendations, or most clinicians will not read them at all. Guidelines should offer clear standards by which to audit: compliance with guidelines may be a valuable part of the process of clinical governance. An example of an innovative approach that has been shown to reduce inappropriate use of fresh frozen plasma (FFP) and platelets, is to combine the transfusion request form with the guidelines [16].

Clinical incident reports and complaints

One important element of clinical governance involves learning from incident reports and from complaints. Complaints are uncommon in transfusion practice, but any mishap or "near miss" should be the subject of an incident report, from which important lessons may be learned (or indeed re-learned). Collecting and analysing clinical incident reports enable recognition of patterns, and identifications of areas and practices associated with special risk.

All staff should share a corporate responsibility for ensuring that their practice complies with their Trust's transfusion policy, but many Trusts have now appointed Transfusion Practitioners (TPs) to monitor compliance and to reflect constructively on lessons learned from critical incident reports. They can also deliver a training programme, under the direction of the HTC (which has the primary responsibility for induction and training programmes for all staff involved in the transfusion process and for setting standards). They are destined to play an increasingly important role in the promotion of good practice, and should be pivotal in the audit and governance of blood transfusion at a local level.

Managing a scarce and costly resource

For Primary Care Trusts clinical governance responsibilities in blood transfusion extend to the commissioning of services that are "safe and value for money in relation to better blood transfusion" [7]. Reducing waste and conserving a scarce resource are therefore important objectives. As in many other areas, Primary Care Trusts had this responsibility thrust upon them when they were inexperienced. So far there are few signs of activity in this area, but hopefully commissioners understand that the quality of support services including blood transfusion have a bearing on the overall delivery of clinical care.

The cost to the hospital blood bank of a unit of red cells in the UK is nominally £117 (2004). The true cost is much higher. A study estimated the annual UK costs of providing and transfusing blood products in 2000/2001 was £898 million, and the estimated cost for an adult red cell transfusion (average 2.7 units) was £635 taking into account both blood transfusion service costs and hospital resource use costs [17].

An important priority of blood bank management is to ensure that the appropriate blood product is available as soon as the decision to transfuse has been made, so allowing demand to be met with smaller stock levels. It is now possible, with a combination of modern rapid matching techniques, electronic issue of blood and efficient stock management, to reduce wastage to negligible levels, but this depends on audit to monitor use and good communications to build up trust and confidence between users and the blood bank. The days when blood was required to be routinely matched in advance, "just in case", have passed. With a shrinking donor pool and rising costs of processing, practices need to be adjusted if the demands of increasing clinical activity are to be met.

Future implications

Until recently, the conservation of blood has hardly registered as an issue on the average clinician's radar. The generosity of donors is taken for granted and in times of shortage donors have always responded to appeals. The time when this may no longer be possible is perhaps approaching. The first report of a possible case of transfusion transmitted variant Creutzfeldt Jakob disease (vCJD) in a human has just been announced [18]. Almost simultaneously we hear of the first case of bovine spongiform encephalopathy (BSE) in the USA. We can speculate on the possible effects of these worrying developments on the world supply of blood and plasma, but we could more usefully review our individual practices and consider changes that could eliminate or reduce the use of allogeneic blood.

Autologous transfusion rates in the UK are low in comparison to those of our European neighbours and the main constraints to increasing use are perceived to be logistical. The removal of these constraints may only result in small increases in individual practice [19]. A strategy to promote autologous techniques is required as well as a catalyst, usually in the form of an enthusiastic surgeon or anaesthetist. Some Trusts are unusually fortunate in having more than one enthusiast, as demonstrated by this manual. With the possibility that concerns about vCJD could have a serious impact on blood supplies, proactive hospital managers and HTCs will already have developed contingency plans giving priority to urgent surgery and operations that do not require blood. A well-organised autologous transfusion service can play a useful role here.

In the next year we can anticipate other developments that will have clinical governance implications. For example, a European Directive [20] may require compliance with new standards in many areas by 2005. Those that will impact on hospital transfusion practice relate to traceability of all blood products from donor to recipient and vice versa, to storage of records for at least 30 years, and to quality management processes. Clinical governance and audit of blood transfusion seem set to dominate the agenda in HTC meetings for years to come.

Key Summary

♦ Blood transfusion practice has been subject to the principles of good audit and governance for many years.

♦ There are now national accreditation schemes for clinical pathology. These and nationally recognised quality control checks are important elements of governance.

♦ National audits have shown variation in blood usage and in the monitoring and delivery of transfusion. These have led to guidelines aimed at reducing unnecessary transfusion and risk.

♦ Hospital Transfusion Committees (HTCs) are responsible for local audit of transfusion practice and for remedying deficiencies (i.e. governance).

♦ Transfusion Practitioners (TPs) will be pivotal in local training and audit.

♦ Clinical incident reports relating to transfusion can provide useful lessons.

♦ A European Directive on traceability of all blood products will have important implications for documentation, record keeping and risk management.

References

1. Department of Health. A First Class Service. Quality in the new NHS. Department of Health, London, 1998.

2. Baglin T. Anticoagulant services - the foundation for clinical governance? *Thrombus* 2003; (7), 3: 5-6.

3. British Committee for Standards in Haematology: In: *Standard Haematology Practice*. Roberts BE, Ed. Blackwell Scientific Publications, Oxford, 1991.
   (a) Code for Good Laboratory Practice in Haematology Laboratories (including Hospital Blood Banks): 1-18.
   (b) Hospital Blood Bank Documentation and Procedures:128-138.
   (c) Product Liability for Hospital Blood Bank: 217-230.
   (d) Implementation of a Maximum Surgical Blood Order Schedule: 189-197.

4. Department of Health. Use of blood for transfusions. *Lancet* 1951; 2: 1044.

5. Grindon AJ, Tomasulo PS, Bergin JJ, *et al*. The hospital transfusion committee. Guidelines for Improving Practice. *JAMA* 1985; 253: 540-543.

6. NHS Executive. Better Blood Transfusion. Department of Health, London, 1998 (Health Service Circular 1998/224).

7. NHS Executive. Better Blood Transfusion: Appropriate Use of Blood. Department of Health, London, 2002 (Health Service Circular 2002/009).

8. British Committee for Standards in Haematology. The administration of blood and blood components and the management of transfused patients. *Transfus Med* 1999; 9: 227-238.

9. Bucknall CE, Ryland I, Cooper A, *et al*. National benchmarking as a support system for clinical governance. *J Roy Coll of Physicians of London* 2000; 34: 52-56

10. Murphy MF, Wilkinson J, Lowe D, *et al*. National audit of the blood transfusion process in the UK. *Transfus Med* 2001; 11: 363-370.

11. Williamson LM, Lowe S, Love EM, *et al*. Serious hazards of transfusion (SHOT) initiative: analysis of the first two annual reports. *BMJ* 1999; 319: 16-19.

12. Sirchia G. For the Sanguis Study Group. Use of blood products for elective surgery in 43 European hospitals. *Transfus Med* 1994; 4: 251-268.

13. Hill SR, Carless PA, Henry DA, *et al*. Transfusion thresholds and other strategies for guiding allogeneic red blood cell transfusion. *Cochrane Database of Systematic Reviews* 2002; (2), CD 002042.

14. Lind M, Vernon C, Cruickshank D, *et al*. The level of haemoglobin in anaemic cancer patients correlates positively with quality of life. *Br J Cancer* 2002; 86 (8): 1243-1249.

15. Cavill I. Reducing blood transfusion. Focus should be on improving patient's ability to make own blood. *BMJ* 2002; 325 (7365): 655.

16. Chang G, Wong HF, Chan A, *et al*. The effects of a self-educating blood component request form and enforcements of transfusion guidelines on FFP and platelet usage. *Clinical and Laboratory Haematology* 1996; 18(2): 83-87.

17. Varney SJ, Guest JF. The annual cost of blood transfusions in the UK. *Transfus Med* 2003; 13: 205-218.

18. Reid J, Secretary of State for Health. Blood transfusion incident involving vCJD. Statement to Parliament, 17 December, 2003.

19. Hill J, James V. Survey of autologous blood transfusion activity in England (2001). *Transfus Med* 2003; 13: 9-15.

20. The European Parliament and the Council of the European Union. Directive 2002/98/EC. *Official Journal of the European Union* (8.2.2003) L33/30-40.

Chapter 22

The Hospital Transfusion Team

Dafydd Thomas MB ChB FRCA

Consultant in Intensive Care and Anaesthesia

Morriston Hospital, Swansea, UK

"... transfusion practices vary quite widely for the same group of patients, undergoing the same or similar operations within the same operating suite."

Introduction

The concept of a Hospital Transfusion Team (HTT) has been outlined in the Health Service Circular *Better Blood Transfusion 2* (BBT2) [1]. As with many successful recipes, not all the secrets are included in the list of ingredients. The success of a Hospital Transfusion Team depends as much on teamwork as on the individual members.

Many Hospital Transfusion Committee (HTC) chairpersons and haematologists involved in transfusion, despair because of the lack of communication between various departments within the hospital. This chapter will attempt to help those of you who are trying to set up a successful hospital transfusion team. It will summarise the factors which may help hospitals develop an enthusiastic and effective team, addressing better clinical blood use within the hospital. The risk of transfusion transmitted disease when using allogeneic blood can never be zero.

Concerns regarding new blood-borne diseases together with changing population demographics are threatening the ability to supply enough blood to meet demand. This further underlines the need to use allogeneic blood in an appropriate manner. The HTT is responsible for promoting this appropriate use of blood.

The role of the HTT

As stated in the HSC 2002/009 [1] the HTT has a role in:

- Assisting in the implementation of the HTC's objectives.
- Promoting and providing advice and support to clinical teams on the appropriate and safe use of blood.
- Actively promoting the implementation of good transfusion practice.
- Supporting the training for all hospital staff involved in the process of blood transfusion.

These points highlight the main aims of a HTT which are to raise awareness amongst staff and very often to change out-dated attitudes to transfusion practice. The success of such a team will depend upon a co-operative approach between the many departments of a hospital. There needs to be a degree of trust within the hospital between the HTT and the various groups of employees that will require education in transfusion matters and allow scrutiny through audit of their practice (Table 1) [2,3]. Many of those clinically involved in transfusion can be persuaded to change practice if the available evidence is provided to support this change. The evidence may be presented in a logical and informative manner at departmental meetings, audit meetings or even through small group discussions.

The transfusion practices that the HTT may call into question have evolved over many years and although judged to be inappropriate by standards today, would have been quite acceptable in the past. A friendly process of education empowers practitioners, making them aware of current thinking. The HTT can act as a stimulus to produce new audit or research material to show that change is of clinical benefit. The greatest achievement of the HTT will be to persuade practitioners that there is a need to change or improve their practice. Once there is a will to embrace change the role of the HTT becomes easy.

Table 1. Comparative audit and the HTT - keys to success.

The usefulness of this audit tool in altering clinical practice should not be underestimated. The essential features are outlined below.

♦ Ensure that information is evidence-based and that you can quote references or examples of best practice.

♦ Audit practice as a baseline.

♦ Allow open discussion at a feedback meeting of audit data.

♦ Try and ensure that the clinicians or healthcare workers being audited have possession of the data and they realise the confidentiality of the audit process.

♦ Always behave with the highest level of integrity and professionalism - this does NOT mean you have to be humourless.

♦ In the instance of less desirable results try and offer encouragement and suggestion about how practice could be improved.

♦ Avoid the generation of a blame culture.

♦ Encourage and praise improvements in practice.

♦ Involve junior staff and persuade the submission of abstracts and poster displays at national or international meetings.

♦ Remember, many people have a competitive side and respond well to comparison, particularly when reported back in a confidential manner.

♦ Ensure that comparison is made against previous performance at an individual level - any improvement is to be encouraged.

Membership of the HTT

The team as outlined in BBT2 consists of some essential members although the importance of encouraging and harnessing enthusiasm is far more important than keeping to a list of desirable appointees. Figure 1 shows the interrelationships between the team and other groups within the hospital, but most importantly, each hospital or Trust needs an enthusiast who will act as a catalyst to begin and perpetuate the reaction between various clinical and laboratory departments. Once an effective team is formed the net result will be a cohesive and logical approach to *Better Blood Transfusion* [1].

Minimal membership includes the lead consultant haematologist for transfusion in the hospital, a hospital transfusion practitioner and a blood bank manager with or without representatives from the HTC. The inclusion of the HTC Chair would be an obvious additional member, but local circumstances may encourage others to join the team, eg. a senior nurse manager or trainee doctors' representative. The HTC is usually chaired by a non-haematologist, entering into the spirit of a hospital-wide transfusion process. The function of the HTT is enhanced if the individuals can be delegated a specific role.

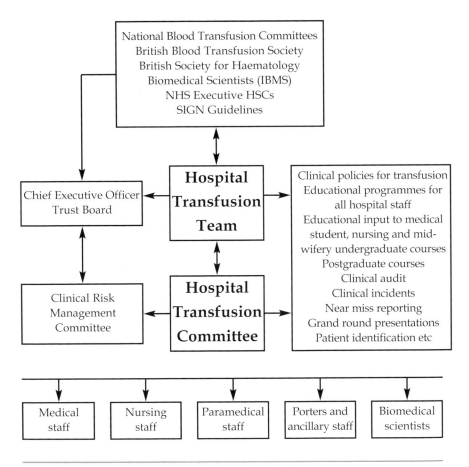

Figure 1 The interrelationships between the HTT, the HTC and other groups within the hospital.

The haematologist

Surprisingly, a special interest in transfusion issues has not always been an essential requirement of hospital-based haematologists. The development of haemato-oncology treatments has overwhelmed the working life of many haematologists, leaving blood transfusion as an area that was considered an uncomplicated and basic part of therapy.

Bleeding and anaemic patients may benefit from allogeneic transfusion. It is true that transfusion will return haematological values to a more normal level, but whether transfusion is always in the patient's best interest is now being called into question. In addition, within the current climate, blood components may not always be readily available, and it is sensible to assess the absolute need for transfusion to enhance what may develop into a rationing of blood component therapy at times of significant shortfall in supply.

The majority of hospitals involve the on-call haematologists in the issue of blood components, especially platelets and fresh frozen plasma (FFP) use [4]. Haematologists are now encouraged to take a more proactive approach and at some larger hospitals there may be a specific consultant who has been delegated the role for transfusion issues.

The blood bank manager

The role of the blood bank manager has expanded to include the audit of blood use within the hospital. Traditionally, there was a requirement to record the blood used as a whole, so that contract volumes could be negotiated with local suppliers. The total number of blood components used would often fluctuate with clinical requirement which is notoriously difficult to predict. More recently, specific audit of clinical usage by subspecialty and even by individual teams or consultants has been available. This information has been used to predict demand more accurately. An additional benefit of audit has been the feedback to individual practitioners on their blood use.

In discussion with the various clinical specialties, the variance in blood component use can be highlighted in a friendly, confidential and nonjudgmental manner [5]. It has been enlightening to see how involved clinicians can become in trying to improve practice and to come into line with other colleagues [6,7,8].

Discussion at departmental and audit meetings may highlight the fact that transfusion practices vary quite widely for the same group of patients, undergoing the same or similar operations within the same operating suite. This information is often enough stimulus to encourage clinicians to examine and change their practice.

The collection of much of these data by the blood bank manager has to-date required painstaking dedication. The use of pathology databases will only act as part of the audit allowing identification of blood issued by requesting surgeon. There are a number of problems with this method of audit. Requests for crossmatch often have the type of operation recorded but without specific detail. For example, there is a huge difference between the blood required for a "nephrectomy". A simple nephrectomy may not require any blood transfusion, whereas a radical nephrectomy for an extensive carcinoma may develop into a major haemorrhage situation. In addition, proof of crossmatch and issue may not mean that the blood has been given. Systems need to be developed that can link with other centrally-held databases, which would allow some assessment of the effect of the blood transfused by recording hospital outcome and length of stay. Hospitals should be encouraged to facilitate this data collection, so that reports can be generated with less effort by the blood bank manager.

Another responsibility of the manager includes the safe issue of blood components from a satellite blood fridge. Poor record-keeping means that time spent out of storage for components not eventually transfused is difficult to ascertain. It remains an important part of clinical audit. Electronic locks requiring bar code identification of the blood component, patient to be transfused and person collecting the blood, can be easily recorded. This technology is available currently but often not in place due to financial constraints. The presence of such systems will not only make the blood bank manager's job easier, it will improve audit accuracy and lead to improved clinical care.

The Transfusion Practitioner (TP)

The Transfusion Practitioner (TP) is a newly created role at the suggestion of the Health Service Circular following the first *Better Blood Transfusion* conference [5]. The full role of the TP is outlined in Chapter 23.

The Chair of the HTC

The success of the HTC depends upon the attendance and co-operation received from the clinicians and managers. The Chair's role is essential to the dynamics of this group. The role requires an impartial approach. It is for this reason that it is recommended that a non-haematologist accepts this position; otherwise it may be perceived that the decrease in blood component use is driven by the financial considerations of the haematology directorate!

It is important that the person appointed is able to encourage debate and persuade individuals to engage in the process of better blood transfusion practice. The attendees at the HTC need to become sufficiently motivated to encourage others within their directorate to address their own practice in the same way.

These individuals have already been mandated by their departments to sit on the HTC and therefore have the trust and backing of that section of the hospital. Their role can be wide ranging but at the very least they can act as a communication link between the HTT, HTC and hospital employees.

The Chair needs to present the case for audit of practice and if necessary, suggest changes to practice where needed. This needs to be done by an inclusive process; authoritative "top-down" approaches will only raise antibodies to change amongst clinicians. To encourage this in a non-threatening atmosphere is essential, allowing the attendees to behave in an adult and confident manner, reassured by the fairness and confidentiality of the process.

The Hospital Transfusion Committee (HTC)

The establishment of a HTC had been considered an integral part of good blood transfusion practice for many years. Despite this, many hospitals either had no such committee or did not have a fully interactive role with many of the end users of blood components.

The BBT1 conference held on the 50th Anniversary of the NHS on July 5th 1998 recommended that all hospitals in the UK should have a HTC. The Committee can encourage a team approach engaging clinicians and laboratory staff in a process of changing transfusion practices, implementing best practice and evidence-based change in outdated clinical beliefs.

Everyone is encouraged to become involved in making and changing policy, dependent on open and active debate at the regular HTC meetings. The HTC should use the summary points highlighted by the Health Service Circular (HSC 2002/009) [1], as its program of action:

♦ Ensure that *Better Blood Transfusion* is an integral part of NHS care.
♦ As part of clinical governance responsibilities, make blood transfusion safer.
♦ Avoid unnecessary use of blood in clinical practice.
♦ Provide better information to patients and the public about blood transfusion.

Priority areas

The main areas that require attention from the HTT and HTC include:

Management awareness

The Chief Executive Officer (CEO) of your hospital may have received both health circulars relating to *Better Blood Transfusion*. An enquiry may have been generated from the CEO's office about what the organisation is doing on the subject, which will have been sent to the Medical Director, and then to the Chair of the hospital's Clinical Risk Management Committee. The query eventually reaches the Chair of the HTC for a reply.

All this assumes that in 1999 when the HSC BBT arrived, that there was a HTC in existence. Certainly by the time BBT2 and Health Service Circular 2001/009 was issued, there should have been the structure of the HTC and Chair in place.

Educating and raising awareness amongst the management support team remains one of the most difficult jobs that the HTT has to perform. Regular reports are required and need to be summarised in the Trust Board's annual report. Any deficiencies in the service need to be outlined and agreement on essential targets for the forthcoming year reached. Current status on implementation of BBT2 needs to be communicated.

The management team needs to be made aware of the European Directive on Blood Transfusion and the legal requirement for vein-to-vein traceability for all blood transfused. The requirement for documentation to be kept for 30 years may sharpen the focus on the problems currently found to be commonplace in the clinical use of blood.

Adequate resources

The team requires adequate support both professionally, managerially and financially [5]. The recommendations in BBT2 for improved blood transfusion have not resulted in any extra monies being made available to Trusts. It is apparent that a business case for a transfusion co-ordinator could be justified if more appropriate transfusion activity resulted in a saving in blood component use; the Trust gaining financially from this improvement in blood transfusion practice.

Regardless of the eventual source of funding for these posts, the HSC outlines a number of areas which will need addressing by the accountants. Individual hospitals have to battle their way through the business case submission that will be required under the current accounting systems. The publication of two HSCs on the topic should lend weight to these submissions.

Improved communication

Good patient care depends upon good communication between the various personnel caring for that patient. All arrangements for admission to hospital and the ordering of specific investigations, drug therapies and planned surgical procedures have set pathways of care which have been well-rehearsed over the years. This may not be the case with new initiatives, as anyone who has tried to implement change within a large organisation knows.

The task of informing hospital carers about a change in practice needs to start with the education of key staff working in many different areas. It is unfortunate that there is reliance on crisis management to give us the opportunity to communicate effectively. When there are acute shortages or when emerging new retrovirus infection reveal themselves it may be too late to try and implement better blood transfusion. The message about blood conservation and appropriate use needs to be sent repeatedly; a warning that there may not be enough blood for everyone that needs it in the future will begin to concentrate minds. This is not an emotive plea. If the plans to increase the availability of joint replacement surgery and myocardial re-vascularisation for all that need it, come to fruition, there will be a great increase in the need for blood transfusion.

The evidence that transfusion is beneficial is not clear, although it is known that bleeding patients die and anaemic patients compromise their tissue oxygen delivery. At what level this becomes critical in the individual is not known, but there is evidence to show that withholding blood transfusion in some groups of patients does not seem to cause harm, and in fact, may be of long-term benefit.

These are the messages that we need to reiterate to our colleagues, encouraging them to audit their practice and allow comparison even in a confidential way with their colleagues, and monitor outcome measures and the effect of transfusion.

This benchmark auditing of practice is an invaluable tool to change practice and needs to be conducted locally, as information from elsewhere will rarely convince distrustful clinicians. In the absence of randomised controlled trials the confidential audit of blood component use is often unexpectedly successful. The audit immediately engages the clinicians in question. They become very interested in the results and will often seek out their own record before the next HTC meeting.

Most audits are carried out retrospectively. This is less time-consuming and will only require a link between the hospital's Patient Administration System and the record of blood given according to the blood bank database. In addition, recording the operation code and treatment given together with hospital discharge status allows a degree of outcome evaluation. The disappointment is that many hospitals are unable to link these databases easily and many audits are painstakingly performed by dedicated blood bank staff with paper and pen! The data is so important that we need to make these tasks more efficient for all concerned.

Critical incident reporting

The HTT is the executive part of the HTC and co-ordinates the clinical transfusion process. The role of optimising pre-operative work-up is highlighted elsewhere. The errors and near miss events related to transfusion is currently part of a confidential reporting system (Serious Hazards of Transfusion [SHOT]), but it is the way in which the HTT responds to these incidents that will make a difference to the safer delivery of blood component transfusion. All incidents need to be investigated so that the errors can be minimised. Critical incidents have familiar patterns and often there are a number of related smaller errors that contribute to these events. Once the mistake has been recognised the individuals need to be interviewed in a non-threatening way. It is important that there is fair blame attached to the incident so that continued reporting occurs. The feedback given to the individuals is often unnecessary as they may already be acutely aware of the mistake. In many instances it is the sheer volume of work that leads practitioners to cut corners on established operating procedures. Sometimes it may be familiarity with an often repeated task which can lead to serious clinical errors. Practitioners need to be encouraged to engage in a period of reflection about the incident (Figure 2). As SHOT has identified consistently, the transfusion of an incompatible component remains the most frequently reported error.

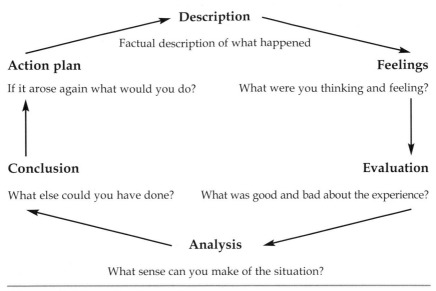

Figure 2. The reflective cycle.

Positive Patient Identification (PPID)

The current systems used for the application of patient identification bands in many hospitals are unsatisfactory. There are various reasons why a patient may be transfused with the wrong blood. These are:

♦ Labelling error of blood component at blood bank.
♦ Labelling error of patient.
♦ Patient ID band removed.
♦ Patient unable to confirm identity.
♦ Error made during the checking procedure due to:

  • lack of knowledge;
  • lack of time;
  • over familiarity with the procedure; and
  • lack of due care and attention to the standard procedures.

It is in this clinical area that the HTT can have its greatest impact, facilitating a safer and better organised approach to clinical transfusion.

The irony about this area of care is that many millions of pounds have been spent on making blood components safer. It is true that these components are now tested more than at any other time, but their use continues to carry risk, and much of this risk occurs in the clinical area where there has been very little investment in education and audit of clinical practice.

Ongoing educational programmes

The HTT and HTC need to establish their authority so that their advice is not only acted upon but actively sought on difficult clinical matters which may be organisational or relate to critical events involving patients.

The need to establish safe policies for transfusion is essential and often requires a well-structured and often repeated programme of lectures and tutorials. As an example, trainee medical staff continue to rotate between a number of hospitals and it may be necessary to have six-monthly refresher tutorials to educate the trainee staff about current policies. This is a role that can be undertaken by any member of the HTT, but increasingly it is falling to the transfusion practitioner.

The HTT, once formed, has a valuable role in facilitating these educational programmes and ensuring that the Trust or hospital has a robust audit system for monitoring both the use of blood components and also their effect - whether positive or negative. This information can then contribute to the national data about variations in transfusion practice. The final link from this national data is to compare the performance of each hospital against a benchmark of best practice and attempt to implement policies that decrease the variance that has been so well-reported in the past.

The benefits to patients are obvious in a system that will ultimately decrease serious clinical errors. Hospitals will benefit financially, not only by the appropriate use of blood components but also by the decreased morbidity and mortality that occur as a result.

Key Summary

◆ Appoint the right people (enthusiastic, independent, friendly, confident team players).

◆ Audit clinical practice.

◆ Operate a "fair blame" culture.

◆ Encourage reflective practice and provide supervisory peer support.

◆ Aim for vein-to-vein documentation and electronic recording of data.

References

1. NHS Executive. Better Blood Transfusion: Appropriate Use of Blood. Department of Health, London, 2002 (Health Service Circular 2002/009).

2. Williams RL, McLellan D, Lees S, Dunlop D. Improving transfusion practices in a busy teaching hospital. *J R Coll Surg Edin* 1997; 42: 314 -16.

3. Shulman IA, lohr K, Derdiaran AK, Picukaric JM. Monitoring transfusionist practices: a strategy for improving transfusion safety. *Transfusion* 1994; 34: 11-15

4. AuBuchon J. The role of transfusion medicine physicians. A vanishing breed? *Arch Pathol Lab Med* 1999; 123: 663-7.

5. AuBuchon JP, Thomas DW. Transfusion Service Management. In: *Transfusion Medicine in Practice,* 2002. Duguid, Goodnough, Desmond, Eds. pp277-292.

6. Scottish Intercollegiate Guidelines Network. Perioperative Blood Transfusion for Elective Surgery - a national clinical guideline. Number 54, October 2001. http://www.sign.ac.uk.

7. The Association of Anaesthetists of Great Britain and Ireland. Blood Transfusion and the Anaesthetist. Red Cell Transfusion, December 2001. http://www.aagbi.org.

8. British Committee for Standards in Haematology, Blood Transfusion Task Force. Guidelines for the clinical use of red cell transfusion. *British Journal of Haematology* 2001; 11: 24-31. http://www.bcshguidelines.com.

Chapter 23

Education in Blood Transfusion and the Transfusion Practitioner

Karen Shreeve RGN RM FETC
Hospital Services Transfusion Practitioner
Welsh Blood Service and Swansea NHS Trust
Elizabeth S Pirie MSc BSc PG Cert RGN
Transfusion Nurse Specialist / Education Co-ordinator, Effective Use of Blood Group,
Scottish National Blood Transfusion Service, Edinburgh, UK

"All hospitals are now required to review their current standards and ensure that local protocols and guidelines are in place for best clinical transfusion practice ...... The Transfusion Practitioner is the key person to deliver this message."

Introduction

The purpose of this chapter is to outline the role of the hospital-based Transfusion Practitioner (TP), thereby aiding those wishing to appoint a suitable candidate and to help consider the training needs of your organisation. Training programmes, whether locally produced or used under licence from an outside agency, can be tailored to meet specific needs as well as the core requirements of national clinical guidelines and government recommendations.

Blood transfusion practice

Blood transfusion is a safe procedure, which, if used appropriately, will save lives or improve quality of life in a large range of clinical conditions. However, safe transfusion practice relies on collaborative teamwork, as blood transfusion is a complex, multi-step process that crosses several professional boundaries and involves many individuals. There are at least 27 stages between taking a blood sample and the recipient receiving their transfusion and there is potential for error at each stage of the process.

The Serious Hazards of Transfusion reporting scheme (SHOT) has demonstrated that in successive years since its launch in 1996, human error has been the major contribution to morbidity and mortality among a significant number of patients receiving blood transfusions [1]. In the seven years of SHOT reporting there have been 1,451 incorrect blood component incidents resulting in 15 deaths and 85 cases of major morbidity. Failure of correct patient or component identification at the time of collection from storage sites and during bedside checking procedures, remain the major cause of these incidents.

Initiatives to improve transfusion practice include the two Health Service Circulars *Better Blood Transfusion* (BBT) [2] and *Better Blood Transfusion 2* (BBT2) [3], which support training and education in transfusion, the introduction of transfusion standards in the Clinical Negligence Scheme for Trusts and guidelines for blood transfusion administration [4]. Forthcoming EC Directives will further impact upon practice with the need to provide "vein-to-vein" traceability [5] and to maintain clinical records of transfusion for 30 years. All hospitals are now required to review their current standards and ensure that local protocols and guidelines are in place for best clinical transfusion practice. All hospital staff involved in the transfusion process should have access to induction and annual mandatory update programmes, which should be supported with up-to-date local policies based on national guidelines (in a similar way to resuscitation or fire lectures).

Each hospital should have a Hospital Transfusion Team consisting of a lead clinician, blood bank manager and transfusion practitioner who will work to support clinical teams in the safe, appropriate and effective use of blood as well as actively promoting good transfusion practice.

The role of the Transfusion Practitioner

A strategy of blood conservation is not complete without clear recognition of the need for allogeneic blood transfusion when it is both safe and clinically appropriate. The TP is seen as the key person to deliver this message [6]. This role has developed in response both to government recommendations and the needs of the service nationally. Their professional background may be scientific, nursing or medical, and he/she has a pivotal role in providing or facilitating transfusion training and education. Another important requirement for the role, whether hospital or regionally based, is the ability to relate to all groups of staff with confidence, from managers and clinicians to ancillary workers. The role of the TP is still evolving and sharing of knowledge and practice is essential for this role. It was with this aim that the peer support group, Specialist Practitioners of Transfusion ("SPOT") was formed, through which a strong communication network now exists. Practitioners benefit from the sharing of knowledge and practice developments accessed via the group's website [7]. At the time of publication there are approximately 170 TPs, some of whom are hospital-based whilst others, employed by the blood centres, fulfil a regional role offering support and guidance to their hospital-based colleagues.

The role of the TP may involve setting up transfusion practice audit, coupled with practice development and education combined with an important responsibility for haemovigilance. There will be variations in the role from region to region, but the following are the main duties of the post:

- Audit and research.
- Training and education.
- Link between hospital transfusion laboratory and clinical areas.
- Increase awareness of current transfusion issues.
- Improve transfusion practice.
- Promote autologous transfusion, in particular cell salvage.
- Encourage the use of alternatives to allogeneic transfusion.
- Ensure the safe and appropriate use of allogeneic blood.
- Investigate transfusion incidents and provide timely feedback to clinical areas.
- Encourage involvement of other staff members in the training process.
- Provide patient information.
- Membership of Hospital Transfusion Committees.
- Ensure multidisciplinary support for transfusion matters.
- Assess clinical transfusion practice (competencies).

The list is not exhaustive and there will almost certainly be other features of the role.

Developing an education programme in hospital-based transfusion practice

Designing and implementing an education programme for transfusion practice that encompasses the diverse staff groups involved in the transfusion process is a challenge. The clinician, phlebotomist, biomedical scientist, porter and the nursing practitioner all have different viewpoints and need to be engaged in the learning process without feeling threatened or patronised. Several methods of programme delivery will need to be considered to allow the essential information to be presented to each of the staff groups.

One of the recommendations from the SHOT report is that all personnel involved in the transfusion process should have their clinical competency assessed. There is increasing interest from educational establishments and employers for proof of clinical competency or at the least a register to ascertain which members have attended the sessions.

To help develop a training programme there are a number of fundamental steps to consider:

- Conduct a training profile and identify the staff groups that will require training.
- Determine in which part of the transfusion process they are involved.
- Identify the person responsible for overall training of each staff group.
- Establish what training is currently provided for each group, at induction and for continuing professional development.
- Note the numbers of potential trainees that the programme would be required to target and work out projected frequency of training sessions and numbers involved with each, to include shift patterns and leave.

Figure 1 shows an example of an adapted training profile derived from these principles [8].

The next step is to undertake an assessment of baseline knowledge and practice within each staff group, followed by a comparison of existing

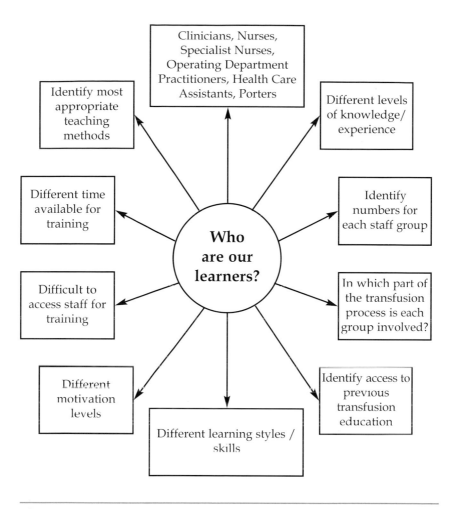

Figure 1. An example of an adapted training profile.

knowledge against the desired standard as set out in the teaching material provided. The level of training required will depend on each staff group and their particular needs so that safe practice is addressed at every level. This sets a challenge for the hospital-based transfusion practitioner given the different knowledge base and scope of practice within each group.

Hospital-based transfusion practice

There are several practical suggestions regarding this preliminary assessment of practice, the development of a training programme and effective communication with all levels of staff involved in the transfusion process.

Local audit

A recent national comparative audit of transfusion practice identified serious shortfalls in knowledge and practice [9]. At every stage of the transfusion process checks are used to minimise the risk to the patient. However, these procedures are meaningless if the operator has insufficient insight as to why checks are made and why errors occur; so, deficits in understanding must be identified and addressed. Also, shortcomings in practice need to be acknowledged so that training programmes can concentrate on local need in addition to the requirements as set out by the regulatory bodies. Areas of knowledge that should be evaluated are as follows:

- Basic blood groups.
- Commonest causes of incompatible transfusion.
- Procedures for blood sampling and labelling.
- Procedures for storage of blood components.
- Collection procedures for blood components.
- Checking and administration procedures for blood components.
- Procedures for monitoring the transfused patient.
- Understanding of adverse events in transfusion.

There are two main methods employed to measure existing knowledge and practice:

- Questionnaire.
- Observation.

Questionnaires should be designed with obligatory standards of practice in mind and will differ for each group of staff. It is useful to include examples of transfusion incidents illustrated in the SHOT reports and ask responders to identify the errors. There are clear disadvantages with this method - for example, poor response rates, deficient completion and the temptation for recipients to give a "correct" rather than realistic response.

Observational audits of transfusion practice can yield a wealth of information; however, they are labour-intensive and are difficult to undertake. Direct observation can make staff alter their practice, but there is evidence to suggest that staff soon become used to the observer and continue with their usual practice [10,11]. Nevertheless, these factors should be taken into account when interpreting the results.

Developing and delivering the programme

Transfusion practice crosses professional boundaries and while there can be much common content in the transfusion education programme, the profile of each group must be taken into account. Developing learning materials requires careful planning and should not be done in isolation. There are advantages in team-working to develop learning materials [12,13]. For example, groups have more skill and knowledge to shape and inform decisions because they can generate a greater variety of ideas and to detect errors. Learning materials should be critically reviewed by a number of subject experts and target users. This will provide the development team with unbiased, objective feedback to ensure that learning materials are designed to take account of each staff group involved in the transfusion process.

The learning needs of each group to be targeted are highlighted below.

Phlebotomists

Phlebotomists are responsible for the majority of routine sampling for pre-transfusion testing. Their core knowledge should include:

- ◆ Knowledge of "sampling incidents" to enhance understanding.
- ◆ The necessity for positive patient identification and correct labelling.
- ◆ Best practice in pre-transfusion compatibility sampling.
- ◆ Basic knowledge of blood groups.

Porters

In many areas porters are key personnel in the transport of blood to the clinical area. Their knowledge base should include:

- ◆ Knowledge of reported "blood collection incidents".
- ◆ The necessity for positive patient and component identification.
- ◆ The correct storage conditions for blood components.
- ◆ Local procedure for collection and delivery of blood components.
- ◆ A practical session on any blood-tracking system in use at the hospital.

Biomedical scientists

Whilst this group has expert knowledge of laboratory practice they may have limited knowledge of the clinical area and the wider elements of the service. Learning needs that have been identified for this group are:

- ◆ Knowledge of the SHOT report.
- ◆ Knowledge of minimum labelling requirements for laboratory samples.
- ◆ Correct entry of patient demographics onto IT systems.
- ◆ Best practice in labelling of blood and components.
- ◆ Basic appreciation of methods of administration of blood and components.
- ◆ Understanding of patient records.
- ◆ Recognition of transfusion reactions.
- ◆ Knowledge of national and European Directives influencing laboratory practice.
- ◆ Practical and theoretical training in the use of any blood-tracking system utilised at the hospital.

Nurses, midwives and operating department practitioners

The personnel within this group may be involved in all stages of the transfusion process and the learning needs to address are:

- ◆ Knowledge of the SHOT report to enhance understanding.
- ◆ Knowledge of basic blood groups and compatibility.

- Informed consent/refusal issues.
- The necessity of positive patient identification at all stages of the transfusion process.
- Best practice in pre-transfusion compatibility sampling and correct labelling.
- How to send routine and emergency blood samples.
- The correct storage conditions for blood components.
- Local procedure for collection and delivery of blood components.
- A practical session on any blood-tracking system in use at the hospital.
- Checking of blood component against the patient.
- How to take initial action to manage an adverse event.
- Awareness of transfusion reactions.
- How to activate the major haemorrhage policy.
- Alternatives to allogeneic transfusion.

Doctors

Clinicians can be involved at almost every point of the transfusion chain, from initiating the transfusion to administering it. They are a "mobile" staff group thereby complicating the delivery of a training programme. Doctors need the core knowledge of the nursing staff and in addition:

- Greater knowledge of blood groups and compatibility.
- Out-of-hours and emergency sampling.
- Ordering of blood components in the routine and emergency situation.
- How to manage an adverse event.
- Management of transfusion reactions.
- Appropriate prescribing in line with protocols and guidelines.

Additionally, each staff group needs to be aware of the unique role of the other groups involved in the transfusion process and how they interact with each other. Some staff will be unable to participate in a collective hospital "induction" or update programme so it may be necessary to deliver education separately to some groups. Various methods can be employed, such as face-to-face teaching programmes, study days, workshops and self-directed learning. Progress is being made with alternative methods of delivery; for example, the Better Blood Transfusion Continuing Education Programme developed by the Scottish National Blood Transfusion Service has recently been launched on an e-learning site www.learnbloodtransfusion.org.uk.

Maintaining momentum

Immediately after training, the staff will demonstrate higher levels of awareness and motivation, but in time this will wane. There are several ways to maintain awareness and motivation across the hospital between training sessions:

- Get to know the staff and maintain a presence.
- Set up a network of "link-nurses" in clinical areas to help disseminate new information and assist with ongoing audit.
- Give early feedback to the site of incidents (eg. from unlabelled or mislabelled samples to the more serious incidents).
- Set up a hospital or Trust Transfusion Team Newsletter (which may be sponsored by appropriate companies, eg. cell salvage, diagnostics, therapeutics).
- Organise "drop-in" sessions with poster displays and lunch.
- Attend departmental audit meetings with current transfusion information.
- Present at the "Grand Round" soon after the medical staff changes.
- Contribute to the doctors' handbook for each firm/speciality.
- Publish web pages on your hospital's intranet.
- Provide *Handbook of Transfusion Medicine* [14] to all clinical areas.
- Design an interactive computer-based training package.

It may also be useful to raise awareness of the following:

- Threats to the future of the blood supply.

  - Demographics, infection, vectors.

♦ Management of the blood supply.

  • Prepared response to shortages, disaster planning.

♦ Alternatives to allogeneic blood.

  • Epoietin.
  • Intravenous iron.
  • Tolerating postoperative anaemia.

♦ Pre-operative optimisation.
♦ Intra-operative cell salvage.
♦ Postoperative wound drain re-infusion.

Conclusions

The document *BBT2* recommends that hospitals minimise the use of allogeneic blood, but as it is unlikely that there will be a substitute to blood transfusion in the foreseeable future, other methods of conservation must be considered. Whilst the theme of this book is blood conservation, allogeneic blood remains a necessity for some and its safe and appropriate use remains the focus of training and education programmes. The SHOT scheme continues to identify shortcomings in current transfusion practice; therefore, it is vital to address the training needs of all staff groups involved in the transfusion process. The TP has a pivotal role to play in planning and co-ordinating training programmes but his/her role may have a wider remit.

We have suggested some basic methods to raise and maintain awareness of current issues in blood transfusion, but there will be many other tactics employed by innovative transfusion practitioners. However, we hope that we have offered guidance and provided the basic ingredients necessary to the newly appointed practitioner.

Key Summary

◆ The Transfusion Practitioner has a pivotal role in education for transfusion practice.

◆ Discover the educational needs of your target groups.

◆ Design your programme to take account of these needs and the specific needs of your hospital.

◆ Use diverse methods of delivery.

◆ Maintain staff awareness of current transfusion issues.

◆ Improve and maintain safety in blood transfusion whether allogeneic or autologous.

◆ Promote use of transfusion alternatives.

References

1.   Stainsby D, Cohen H, Jones H, *et al.* Serious Hazards of Transfusion: Annual Report, 2001-2002. Serious Hazards of Transfusion Steering Group, Manchester, 2003.

2.   NHS Executive. Better Blood Transfusion. Department of Health, London 1998 (Health Service Circular 1998/224).

3.   NHS Executive. Better Blood Transfusion: Appropriate Use of Blood. Department of Health, London 2002 (Health Service Circular 2002/009).

4.   Murphy MF, Atterbury CLJ, Chapman JF, *et al.* The administration of blood and blood components and the management of transfused patients. *Transfus Med* 1999; 9: 227-238.

5.   EC. Directive 2002/98/EC of the European Parliament and of the Council of 27 January 2003. Setting standards of quality and safety for the collection, testing, processing, storage and distribution of human blood and blood components and amending Directive 2001/83/EC. 2003.

6.   Gray S, Melchers RA. Transfusion Nurses - the way forward. In: Serious Hazards of Transfusion: Annual Report, 2000-2001. Serious Hazards of Transfusion Steering Group, Manchester, 2002.

7.   Shreeve K, McCart T. www.bloodspot.org.

8.   Rowntree D. *Preparing materials for open, distance and flexible learning.* Kogan Page, London, 1994.

9.   Stainsby D, Murphy MF, Regan F, *et al.* National Comparative Audit of Blood Transfusion, 2004. National Blood Service and the Royal College of Physicians.

10.   Whitsett CF, Robichaux MG. Assessment of blood administration procedures: problems identified by direct observation and administrative incident reporting. *Transfusion* 2001; 41: 581-586.

11.   Kaplan H. Lessons learned. *Transfusion* 2001; 41: 575-576.

12.   Race P, Brown S. *500 Tips for teachers.* Kogan Page, London, 1993.

13.   Ellington H, Percival F, Race P. *A handbook of educational technology.* 3rd ed. Kogan Page, London, 1993.

14.   McClelland DBL. *Handbook of Transfusion Medicine.* 3rd ed. The Stationery Office, London, 2001.

Chapter 24

Regulatory Framework

Virge James DM (Oxon) FRCPath MBA
Consultant Haematologist, National Blood Service, Sheffield, UK
Dorothy Stainsby FRCP FRCPath
Consultant Haematologist, National Blood Service, Newcastle upon Tyne, UK

"The regulatory framework impacting on blood conservation is complex."

Introduction

The rules, regulations, guidelines and initiatives covering blood conservation techniques emanate from many sources. For simplicity they can be considered under the following headings:

♦ European Union.
♦ Council of Europe.
♦ National.
♦ Professional organisations.
♦ Patient networks including Jehovah's Witnesses.
♦ International.

The list is not exhaustive, and inevitably some overlap will occur. In this short chapter we provide a brief overall summary and refer the reader to the publication or website for more detailed information.

European Union (www.europa.int)

There are now 25 Member States in the European Union. The EU issues Regulations, Directives and Recommendations. Regulations and Directives have the force of law.

Several EU Directives are relevant but it must be emphasised that the EU has no jurisdiction on how Member States' health services are run or on clinical practice [1].

♦ EU Directive 2002/98/EC *Setting standards of quality and safety for the collection, testing, processing, storage and distribution of human blood and blood components* sets out legally binding regulations for blood establishments (blood services) and hospital blood banks. The Directive impacts on blood conservation in a number of ways: it requires haemovigilance, i.e. reporting of carefully defined serious adverse events and reactions related to blood transfusion to a designated "Competent Authority"; it requires full traceability of all blood components; it defines Predeposit Autologous Donation (PAD) and stipulates that the same regulations apply to PAD as to allogeneic blood. This Directive will be incorporated into legislation in February 2005. At the time of writing the Competent Authority for most countries has not been determined.

This Directive does not cover other forms of autologous transfusion as these are part of clinical practice. It also does not cover non-remunerated blood donation which is essential to maintain the safest source of blood and retain high ethical standards.

♦ A series of three Directives regulating the safety and marketing of medical devices throughout the EU came into effect from 1 January 1993 [2]. These Directives benefit both patients and industry. They set out essential requirements that products must meet and thus harmonise controls within a single system avoiding the need for manufacturers to comply with 25 different sets of rules. Devices meeting these requirements are generally CE marked to indicate compliance. There are a few exceptions.

The definition of a medical device is extensive and all instruments and equipment used in blood conservation, including the software involved, are covered by this definition.

♦ The Medical Devices Regulations 2002 [3] consolidate all the existing regulations into a single piece of legislation and came into effect on 13 June 2003.

CE marking applies to electrical and technical standards and not to the clinical performance of the device or the quality of the blood product. In the UK, the National Institute for Clinical Excellence has instituted a programme (Health Technology Assessment) responsible for the regulation and introduction of novel devices (see below).

Council of Europe (www.coe.int)

The CoE has been active in promoting voluntary blood donations in all its Member States (currently 45 and including all EU members) and has since 1995 produced *A Guide to the Preparation, Use and Quality Assurance of Blood Components*. This publication is revised annually by several groups of experts. The 10th Edition was published in 2004 (ISBN 92-871-5393-0) and Chapter 20 of this publication covers autologous predeposit transfusion.

The European Union and Council of Europe are independent, but the CoE guide forms the basis of the more detailed technical requirements of the EU Directive. National experts advise the CoE and, therefore, influence the contents of the guide and the Directive.

National

Better Blood Transfusion (www.gov.uk)

Although the UK is one Member State in the EU and also in the CoE, since 1991 there are four devolved governments and the Health Service functions differently in each. The Chief Medical Officers of all four countries participated in a conference in October 2001 and signed up to the national Directive Health Service Circular (HSC) 2002/009 *Better Blood Transfusion*, although separate variations of the circular have been issued:

- ◆ Welsh Health Circular WHC (2002) 137, issued by the Welsh Assembly Government http://cymruweb.wales.nhs.uk.
- ◆ NHSHDL (2003) 19 Scottish Executive.
- ◆ HSS (MD) 6/03 Northern Ireland.

To all intents and purposes they are the same but the manner of implementation varies. There is an expectation that both the Healthcare Commission and Clinical Negligence Scheme for Trusts (qv) will require Trusts to provide evidence of efforts to achieve implementation of this guidance.

All four national blood/blood transfusion services are actively promoting the implementation of this HSC, known as BBT2, and have produced or are producing strategies for the conservation of donor blood

The strategy for England, produced by a multidisciplinary team from all four countries, has been sent to the National Blood Transfusion Committee who together with the Department of Health in England are planning implementation. The main elements of this strategy suggest concentrating efforts on:

- Education.
- Audit.
- Pre-assessment for elective surgery.
- Intra-operative cell salvage.

National regulatory bodies

Medicines and Healthcare Products Regulatory Authority (MHRA) (www.mhra.gov.uk)

The MHRA was created in 2002 by the fusion of the Medicines Control Agency and Medical Devices Agency. It is the Competent Authority for the UK blood services. The Competent Authority is the body responsible for implementing the requirements of the Directives in each Member State. The MHRA's main role is to ensure that the manufacturers comply with the Regulations. It is also authorised to inspect and licence blood establishments (blood services) and tissue banks.

The Healthcare Commission (HCA) (www.chai.org.uk)

This organisation replaces the work of the Commission for Health Improvement and has also taken over some responsibilities from the National

Care Standards Commission for the voluntary and private sectors, and from the Audit Commission relating to cost-effectiveness of healthcare. It exists to promote improvement in quality of healthcare in England and Wales and will undertake inspections of implementation of NICE guidance and National Service Frameworks. It will also investigate serious service failures and will commission and support national clinical audits.

The NHS Litigation Authority (NHSLA) (www.nhsla.com)

This Authority is a special health authority which indemnifies NHS bodies in respect of both clinical negligence (the Clinical Negligence Scheme for Trusts) and non-clinical risks, and manages claims and litigation under both headings. The NHSLA also has risk management programmes in place against which NHS Trusts are assessed.

Professional guidelines, databases and sytematic reviews

Guidelines

Almost all "learned societies" have produced guidelines on blood conservation methods:

- British Committee for Standards in Haematology www.bcshguidelines.com.
- Association of Anaesthetists www.aagbi.org.
- Clinical Effectiveness and Evaluation Unit of the Royal College of Physicians www.rcplondon.ac.uk/college/ceeu/ceeu_guidelinedb.asp.
- The UKBTS/NIBSC Joint Professional Advisory Committee. This is a variable body of experts from numerous disciplines and produces the *Guidelines for the UK Blood Transfusion Services and the Handbook of Transfusion Medicine*. The 4th Edition of the latter is expected in 2004. Both are available on www.transfusionguidelines.org.uk.

National Institute for Clinical Excellence (NICE) (www.nice.org.uk)

The National Institute for Clinical Excellence was set up as a special health authority for England and Wales on 1 April 1999. It is part of the

National Health Service (NHS), and its role is to provide patients, health professionals and the public with authoritative, robust and reliable guidance on current "best practice". The guidance covers both individual health technologies (including medicines, medical devices, diagnostic techniques, and procedures) and the clinical management of specific conditions.

An assessment of the use of erythropoietin in chemotherapy-induced anaemia is in preparation (due November 2005) and a guideline on anaemia in renal failure is due in 2006.

NICE has established a number of National Collaborating Centres (NCCs) to harness the expertise of the Royal Medical and Nursing Colleges, professional bodies and patient/carer organisations when developing clinical guidelines. Each centre is a professionally-led group with the experience and resources to develop guidance for the NHS on behalf of NICE.

NICE funds three organisations that undertake research into the way patients are treated, to identify ways of improving the quality of care. These organisations are known as National Confidential Enquiries, or "Enquiries" for short. Relevant to blood conservation is *The National Confidential Enquiry into Patient Outcome and Death (NCEPOD)* which examines the outcomes of patients who have received a surgical or medical intervention.

The Confidential Enquiries publish reports summarising key findings and recommendations arising from the information they gather. They aim to identify changes in clinical practice that will improve quality of care and ultimately improve patient outcomes.

Health Technology Assessment (HTA) (www.hta.nhsweb.nhs.uk)

The HTA programme is a national programme of research established and funded by the Department of Health's research and development program.

The HTA commissions assessments of new technology. An assessment of cost-effectiveness of cell salvage and alternative methods of minimising peri-operative allogeneic blood transfusion is in preparation.

Systematic reviews

The Cochrane collaboration can be most easily accessed via the National Electronic Library for Health (www.nehl.nhs.uk). Several relevant systematic reviews are in progress.

The Scottish Intercollegiate network www.sign.ac.uk has produced guidelines on peri-operative cell salvage.

National databases

There are many national databases set up by professional organisations, collecting outcome data for specialties and procedures, such as the National Vascular Database, the National Adult Cardiac Surgical Database and the National Joint Registry. All include data related to blood transfusion and clinical outcome. The current problem is that of meshing data between the various systems in the absence of a unified national patient record system.

Monitoring and learning from adverse events

Serious Hazards of Transfusion (SHOT) (www.shotuk.org)

The SHOT scheme was launched in November 1996 and is a confidential reporting system, voluntary until implementation of the EC Directive in February 2005. SHOT collects data on serious adverse events of transfusion of blood components and makes recommendations aimed at improving transfusion safety. Over 90% of UK hospitals participate in SHOT and successive reports have highlighted the importance of avoidable errors in the transfusion process. Adverse events associated with PAD and the re-infusion of autologous blood should be reported to

SHOT. If this also involves a defect in a blood salvage device this should be reported to the MHRA.

National Patient Safety Agency (NPSA) (www.npsa.nhs.uk)

The NPSA is a special health authority created in July 2001 to co-ordinate efforts in England and Wales to report, and more importantly, to learn from mistakes and problems that affect patient safety. To achieve this aim it has embarked on a training programme in root cause analysis for NHS staff and has established a network of Patient Safety Managers. The NPSA seeks to promote an open and fair culture in the NHS, encouraging all healthcare staff to report incidents without undue fear of personal reprimand. It plans to collect reports throughout the country and initiate preventative measures. The NPSA does not duplicate or replace SHOT and MHRA, but aims to work in collaboration to improve blood transfusion safety.

Patient networks including Jehovah's Witnesses
(www.watchtower.org)

The empowerment of patients has led to many patient organisations and the production of information leaflets by self-help groups. The importance of the internet in providing both valuable and misleading information cannot be underestimated. The most co-ordinated and successful international effort has been that of Jehovah's Witnesses. They produce educational literature and videos of high quality. All are available from their Hospital Liaison Committee network.

International

The Canadian Co-ordination Office for Health Technology Assessment www.ccohta.ca produces clear summaries of international activity in the field of blood transfusion. The International Study of Perioperative Transfusion (ISPOT) organisation has produced powerful comparative data to encourage the appropriate use of transfusion www.lri.ca/programs/ceu/ispot/default.htm. The American Association of Blood Banks has a web presence with excellent information and useful hyperlinks www.aabb.org.

Conclusions

The regulatory framework impacting on blood conservation is complex. It is hoped that professionals, patients, industry and governments can all work together to promote blood conservation thus reducing the risk of inappropriate transfusions to patients.

Key Summary

◆ National guidelines for blood administration have been issued.

◆ Guidelines have also come from learned societies and professional organisations.

◆ Which of the above guidelines should take precedence is unclear.

◆ The European blood Directive is the first EC legislation covering blood components.

- The Directive is binding and must be translated into members' legislation.
- Clinical blood transfusion practice is not covered.

References

1. Duncan B. Health policy in the European Union, how it is made and how to influence it. *BMJ* 2002; 324: 1027-1030.

2. www.mhra.gov.uk.

3. The Medical Devices Regulations, 2002 (SI 2002/618; ISBN 011042317).